The Ginger Book

THE ULTIMATE HOME REMEDY

Stephen Fulder, Ph.D.

Avery Publishing Group

Gar New York

D1468966

This book has been written and published strictly for informational purposes, and in no way should it be used as a substitute for recommendations from your own medical doctor or healthcare professional. All the facts in this book came from medical files, clinical journals, scientific publications, personal interviews, and the personal-practice experiences of the authorities quoted or sources cited. You should not consider the educational material herein to be the practice of medicine or to replace consultation with a physician or other medical practitioner. The author and publisher are providing you with the information so that you can have the knowledge and can choose, at your own risk, to act on that knowledge.

Cover designer: William Gonzalez
In-house editor: Elaine Will Sparber
Typesetter: Bonnie Freid
Printer: Paragon Press, Honesdale, PA

Library of Congress Cataloging-in-Publication Data

Fulder, Stephen.
    The ginger book : the ultimate home remedy / Stephen Fulder.
    p. cm.
    Includes index.
    ISBN 0-89529-725-6
    1. Ginger—Therapeutic use. I. Title.
RM666.G488F85 1996
615'.32421—dc20   95-51401
                                      CIP

Printed in the United States of America.

10 9 8 7 6 5 4 3 2 1

Contents

Acknowledgments

The author would like to thank above all the late John Blackwood, who collected historical and other material for the book, assisted in the writing of the historical section, and reviewed the manuscript. Thanks are also due David Roser and Alan Clements, for their support and encouragement.

The author is grateful to Dr. James A. Duke of the U.S. Department of Agriculture, Beltsville, Maryland, for his table of biologically active compounds in ginger. He would also like to acknowledge his debt to Charles Seely, author of *Ginger Up Your Cookery* (London: Hutchinson Benham, 1982), for several recipe ideas that were adapted for this book.

Preface

We know what a drug is—or, at least, we think we know. A drug is a pure chemical compound that treats a specific disease. It costs hundreds of thousands of dollars to develop and test, and it is supposed to perform "miracles" for us, although there is a fair chance that it will also have adverse effects. These are relatively new beliefs, however. For all of human history before the twentieth century, a medicine was regarded as something else—a plant, made into a tea or extract, that is mild and safe, that does not perform instant miracles but can nevertheless be used to treat every kind of health problem, and that is part of tradition and culture.

Until very recently, we had been ignoring the immense storehouse of healing knowledge accumulated by our ancestors. We are now beginning to reawaken, however. We are realizing that many drugs are more toxic than we originally thought; that many, such as anti-inflammatory drugs for asthma and eczema, do not actually cure disease but just suppress symptoms. It is becoming evident that many drugs are a huge drain on our resources. Today, one-third of Americans are using alternative medicines, the herb industry is booming, remedies such as garlic are becoming top sellers in neighborhood drug stores, and the pharmaceutical industry is scrambling to find new medicines from plants. We are suddenly remembering that most drugs came from plants in the first place and that they were a lot safer in their original God-given plant package.

Against this backdrop, I decided to write a book on ginger. I chose ginger because it is simply one of the most important home remedies on this planet. In the Asian world, billions of people use ginger as an essential part of daily life, valuing it as an important medicine. They believe that ginger saves lives and relieves many uncomfortable symptoms. According to studies, ginger is an effective medicine for stomach upsets, nausea, and vomiting. It cleans the body of toxins. It combats all kinds of infections, especially chronic infections that do not want to clear up. It awakens the immune system and the body's defenses. It fights arthritic complaints and circulatory problems. It helps the system absorb other foods and medicines. It warms the body. And it does all of these things in complete safety. At the same time, ginger is a delicious flavoring that adds a spicy interest to almost any dish.

For most people in the West, however, ginger is merely the tangy taste in ginger beer and ginger cookies. Westerners generally view the intense use of ginger as a medicinal food as a bizarre practice. Yet with half the world relying on ginger so extensively, are we Westerners missing something? This book is my answer to that question.

In this book, I will focus mostly on how ginger can be brought back into daily family health care. I will discuss in detail how ginger can help maintain the digestive system and treat digestive upsets, how it can help keep the circulation in good shape, and how it can help ward off or treat infections and other health problems. To do this, I will draw on the wealth of traditional knowledge handed down by our ancestors, backing up those beliefs with modern science whenever possible. I will also discuss the ginger plant in all its glory, explain how it is grown and processed, and examine the sources of its aroma, taste, and medicinal effects. Since the history and folklore of ginger are fascinating, I will also present stories about ginger's power in traditional village life, especially in India, and of its role in the spice trade, in European and Middle Eastern history, and in herbalism. Finally, I will not forget cooks, rounding out my presentation with recipes and suggestions on how to "ginger up" the diet.

I will discuss ginger in this book as a *spice* and as a *medicinal food*. But first, I would like to briefly define those terms. *Spices* are aromatic seeds, barks, or roots, coming mostly from hot climates and used to flavor foods. They include everything from anise and cardamom to mustard and turmeric. *Herbs*, too, often contain aromatic constituents and are used both as flavorings and medicines. Examples are bay leaf, mint, rosemary, and sage. But herbs differ from spices in that they are mostly leaves and hail from temperate climates.

Medicinal foods are foods that contain, besides nutritional components, special components that have therapeutic effects on our bodies. Of course, this is not a hard and fast definition, since nutritional components such as beta-carotene, found in vegetables, can also be therapeutic. However, the importance of medicinal foods such as licorice, garlic, and ginger lies in their constituents of glycyrrhizin, allicin, and gingerol, respectively, which have purely medicinal, non-nutritive roles in our lives.

Hopefully, by the time you reach the end of this book, you will have begun to understand and "feel" ginger as a good friend and ally. Hopefully, you will bring ginger back into your kitchen and medicine cabinet. Then, when you have realized the true nature and possibilities of this one plant, you will try other plants, too, to enrich your health, your experience, and your life.

As they fell from heaven, the plants said, "Whichever living soul we pervade, that man will suffer no harm."

—*Rig-Veda*

CHAPTER 1

Ginger as Medicine

Most of us have learned during our lives to rely on "modern medicine." In fact, many of us feel that we owe our lives to it, since doctors of one sort or another—obstetricians, pediatricians, general practitioners, internists, gynecologists, geriatricians, and a dozen or so more—follow us every step of our way. But sometimes, it also seems as if nature, which is certainly the first and best physician, has been left in the shadows, upstaged (perhaps unintentionally) by the medical profession.

This is how things stand today in the Western world. But elsewhere—in Central and South America, China, India, and other faraway places—people still live close to nature and know how to use nature's resources to keep themselves well and to treat illness.

A NEW LOOK AT OLD REMEDIES

Like all children, those in my family fall prey to the usual childhood ailments. They have fevers, aches and pains, sore throats, colds, stomach upsets, headaches, illnesses such as measles, and so on. This is a natural process, the body's way of learning about sickness and how to fight it. But when my children fall ill, my wife and I do not automatically react the way most of today's parents do—that is, we do not immediately call the doctor to get a prescription in the belief that the key to health lies mainly in taking the right medication.

Instead, my wife and I simply go into the garden for some fresh herbs, or into the kitchen for some dried herbs or spices, then make a tea or similar therapeutic concoction to give to the sick child as appropriate. If the child has an infection, we might try a fruit diet for a couple of days. We might also employ such proven methods for reducing symptoms as wet towels to bring down a fever or a chest massage with warm olive oil to reduce a cough. We use remedies that have been tested for thousands of years and found to be reliable and safe.

Since my wife and I are not medical practitioners, if a health problem looks unusual or serious, we seek advice from a local holistically minded doctor. We ask the doctor questions, particularly about whether the ailment is "self-limiting"—that is, whether the body can be expected to throw off the affliction by itself. We ask whether the medical treatment suggested is curative or treats only the symptoms. We usually are appreciative of the information and reassurances but find we do not need the prescriptions. Fortunately, over the past two decades, since we first started becoming familiar with natural remedies, we have hardly ever had to take any medications. Moreover, when our children become sick, the illness tends to be mild and run its course quickly. Nor do the children suffer the same ailment again and again, as happens so often with problems such as stomach upsets, cystitis, bronchitis, and ear infections.

Some people might say that my children have genetic superhealth. This may be true, but it is unlikely—they do become sick, after all. Rather, I am convinced that most children would be strong and well, with effective immune systems, if they were provided with the following basics:

- Natural care, meaning breast-feeding during infancy, followed by a nutritious diet, clean water, a healthy environment, lots of exercise, and a minimum of junk foods such as soft drinks, processed foods, and empty snacks. Natural care is not the subject of this book, but one or two good sources of information are given in "Further Reading," page 131.

- A secure emotional and physical environment.

- Safe remedies that work with our natural healing powers when we are ill. Ginger is one such remedy.

At this point, you may say, "It is all well and good for the experts to treat themselves with these remedies, but can ordinary people also rely on them?"

Of course we can. The fact is that people have been treating themselves for common ailments with the plants and remedies around them since the beginning of human history. The knowledge of how to do so used to be cultural—that is, it was learned automatically, just as today's children learn as a matter of course how to switch on the lights and change the channel on the television. Ordinary people used to learn about hawthorn and horehound the same way that we now learn about IBM PC and Macintosh computers.

Today, with most of herbal lore and knowledge lost to us, we feel insecure about using herbs and spices when we are faced with sickness. However, we can gradually relearn how to employ them and, as we do, apply them more and more. Our degree of success will depend on our level of knowledge. The more we know, the more confident we will be at treating simple health problems ourselves with the materials at hand. My purpose in writing a whole book on one spice is to help bring this awareness back into circulation, to restore one more item of our lost inheritance, and to provide us with one more safe tool for self-care.

WHEN CAN HERBS AND SPICES HELP?

It is important to consider to what extent household remedies such as ginger can be used in place of a visit to the doctor. First, we should remember that doctors never see most of our passing symptoms. Research has shown that three-quarters of all incidents of ill health, such as headaches and stomach upsets, are handled at home, mostly by doing nothing. Clearly, therefore, if we stock up on a few good herbal weapons and the knowledge of how to use them, we will only gain.

Second, whenever an illness hangs on, has strong or debilitating symptoms, is raging out of control, or is mysterious in nature, you should not hesitate to see your medical practitioner and get a proper diagnosis. Self-treatment is appropriate only for the kinds of mild, nondangerous health problems we discuss in this book, most of which eventually clear up by themselves.

Third, many of these minor health problems or symptoms are not curable by a doctor anyway, so we have nothing to lose by trying herbal treatments. For example, influenza is a viral disease that does not respond to any modern medicine, although there are medications, such as acetaminophen, that make the illness more bearable. Natural remedies can do the same.

Fourth, no conflict exists between professional help and

self-care. You can do both at the same time. In fact, a good doctor will encourage you to assist in looking after yourself during an illness to lessen your dependence on medications and to help you recover more quickly.

FOODS AS MEDICINES

It may seem strange to pop into your kitchen for your medicine rather than to drive to the local pharmacy. This is because most people assume that foods cannot also be medicines and that even if a certain food does have some action on the body, that action is too weak to make a noticeable difference. However, certain food components are, in fact, the best medicines because they are so safe. Foods certainly can have effects on the body beyond providing carbohydrates, fats, proteins, and vitamins. Just look at the sheer dynamite of a teaspoonful of chili powder for proof of how powerful plant foods can be.

When we look at food, we normally look just at nutritional value. But plants have many other interesting components waiting to be discovered and used. These include flavorings, aromatics, colorings, and chemicals that the plant makes to, for example, protect itself from insects or help control its growth. All of these components can also have a medicinal, non-nutritional effect on us. At the very least, these extra plant substances can prevent illness. One example is cancer. Most cancer experts now agree that green, yellow, and orange vegetables and fruits can help prevent this dread disease. The minerals, fiber, and oily components such as beta-carotene appear to be responsible. The National Cancer Institute of the National Institutes of Health is investing $20 million in a "designer foods" program to learn which protective substances can be added to common staple foods to make them cancer preventives. These substances are being sought in plants such as garlic, flax seed, citrus-fruit extracts, rosemary, and licorice, all of which have both nutritional and medicinal uses.

Again, one of the reasons people assume that food is not medicine is modern society's ignorance. We are taught in childhood that illness is treated with medications, which have strong and more or less immediate effects on the body. Most medications are pure chemicals sold as little pills. Yet for thousands of years, food substances—especially plants such as mint, turmeric, garlic, onion, lemon, and ginger— were acknowledged to be highly effective medicines. While living in India, I was struck by the fact that, in many local households, the mother prepared spice mixtures and the day's recipes according to how each member of the family felt, the weather, the season, and any special weaknesses or vulnerabilities within the family. A household member with arthritic problems, for example, would get bitter foods, with hot spices such as chili, ginger, and pepper. Someone with poor digestion would be given foods with aromatic seeds such as aniseed, coriander, and fennel, as well as mild lentil soups. This is common folk wisdom. The professionals in traditional medicines such as Ayurveda in India and Oriental medicine in China have developed this into a science, with elaborate systems for both preventing and treating ailments with food components.

THE POWER OF SPICES

A good deal of ignorance exists about the real power of spices and, indeed, about why spices were ever used at all. For example, we learned in school that spices were introduced into the diet for the sole purpose of preserving food in hot climates. In medieval times, we were taught, poor folk put ground cumin over meat before hanging it because they did not enjoy the benefit of refrigeration.

The truth is that spices were an amazing discovery. Adding them to food achieves a range of very valuable results, of which food preservation is one but by no means the most important or the most interesting. Spices are used because:

- They are concentrated sources of valuable nutrients, especially vitamins and minerals. For example, garlic has the highest concentration of selenium of any known food plant, and tamarind has exceedingly high levels of vitamin C.

- They help make foods more easily digestible. For example, ginger has been found to contain high levels of the enzymes that break down meat, just as the enzymes in the stomach do. Therefore, ginger acts as a meat tenderizer.

- They help the entire digestive system to function better and to absorb foods better. For example, pungent spices, such as black pepper and ginger, stimulate circulation in the intestine and aid absorption of the other food components of a meal. Spices such as aniseed and cumin calm the stomach and aid the digestive process. Many spices help elimination—flax seed is a mild laxative, and garlic helps the system to excrete fat and cholesterol.

- They can stimulate the appetite, as well as increase the flow of saliva and digestive juices. For example, fenugreek and nutmeg are appetite stimulants.

- They can act as food preservatives. For example, turmeric and cumin seed can help prevent food from spoiling.

- They are antioxidants. For example, rosemary, ginger, and bay-leaf extracts have been found to be as strong as modern chemical antioxidants. They help prevent rancidity and the development of "off" flavors.

- They have an important ability to balance out the general physiological results of a particular diet. For example, the Indian vegetarian diet can be too "cooling," encouraging cold-type ailments such as arthritis and bronchial conditions. Spices can warm the diet to create a healthy energetic balance.

- They correct distortions in individual diets. For example, too many beans can cause flatulence, which can be prevented with asafetida, a medicinal plant resin; too much fat can cause obesity and circulatory problems, which can be prevented with onions and garlic; too much starch can cause tiredness or blood-sugar imbalance, which can be prevented with fenugreek; and too much fruit can cause mucus, which can be prevented with cardamom.

- They detoxify the body and help eliminate poisons that may have contaminated food. For example, cayenne pepper causes poisons to be sweated out, garlic neutralizes toxins in the tissues, and turmeric helps eliminate poisons from the liver.

All of these properties are in addition to the specific medicinal effects of spices. Culinary and aromatic herbs have uses similar to those of spices.

THE RENAISSANCE OF MEDICINAL FOODS

With such a catalogue of benefits, spices would be a worthwhile addition to our diet even if they tasted downright horrible. What a pleasant surprise, then, to find that they add so much to the flavor and aroma of food. It is like having our cake and eating it too. But maybe this is not accidental. Maybe human consciousness is designed in such a way that these beneficial agents are interpreted as pleasing to the senses. Or perhaps the spices themselves are designed to be pleasing. Most likely, however, everything is designed for mutual benefit and interaction. This is certainly something worth mulling over as you cut a piece of ginger to rescue your stomach and the room fills with its full, spicy, exotic aroma.

Not so long ago, many herbs, spices, and other plants were in all the Western *pharmacopoeias* (official drug guides). At the beginning of this century, you could find in these books syrup of ginger, oil of rosemary, dill water, syrup of figs, thyme oil or extract, peppermint oil, and many others. These natural remedies were eventually replaced with stronger chemical preparations, without any testing to see whether the new agents were actually more effective than the old. The old remedies were discarded simply because they did not fit into the scientific way of thinking. Only now are we recognizing that modern medicines carry unexpected and unacceptable price tags—they drain both our wallets and our long-term health and well-being.

But the times are changing. We are witnessing a dramatic renewal of interest in medicinal foods. In 1992, for example, the fastest selling over-the-counter remedy in Europe for the cardiovascular system was garlic, taken in capsules or tablets by 5 million people every day. In 1991, garlic was the most popular of all the remedies available in pharmacies in Germany. At least $100 million worth is sold annually in the United States. Other natural remedies—such as mint, alfalfa, carrot oil, rosemary, cranberry, black currant seed, and thyme—are now also becoming available in all health-food outlets. Ginger, too, is taking off as a health supplement, and it is the purpose of this book to explain how to get the best out of it.

Obvious questions still remain to be answered. When are herbs and spices foods and when are they medicines? How do you take them as medicines compared to consuming them as foods? And are they strong enough when combined with other ingredients during cooking to have real medicinal powers?

The answers never can be absolutely clear-cut because these substances are foods and medicines simultaneously. However, you can imagine that if you put a pinch of curry powder that has been sitting in your cupboard for years into a whole pot of vegetables and cook the mixture furiously, the minimal spicy constituents of the curry powder will be unlikely to have any medicinal effects on your body. Similarly, if you put three drops of clove oil onto an infected tooth and the pain subsides almost immediately, you can hardly call this a culinary experience. Most cases fall somewhere in between.

In general, if you add spices to food, the spices will have a mildly preventive effect against disease, the degree of which will depend on how much of the spice you put in and how much degradation takes place during cooking. If you put in enough to produce a strong taste, you can be sure that most of the physiological effects described in the list on pages 7–8 will occur, especially if you use spices on a regular basis in your diet. On the other hand, if you wish to achieve a specific medicinal result, you should take the spice separately, not as an ingredient in a food dish, and in a prescribed quantity. That way, you will know you are getting the full dosage. In addition, a sensible precaution is to take a medicinal food as a specifically designed medicinal product. Food products may be weak, impure, old, or lacking a sufficient quantity of the medicinal ingredient. In other words, you can choose either the medicinal or the nutritional aspect of a plant by selecting the dose and the manner in which you take it.

WHY GINGER?

There is more to ginger than meets the eye. Once I had a viral infection and a mid-range fever that seemed to drag on and on. I was feeling wretched—restless, achy, hot inside, and constantly nauseous, with an awful headache and difficulty sleeping—the kind of misery that you think will never end when you are in the middle of it but that is soon forgotten when you recover. I asked for a strong ginger tea, made from grated fresh ginger and honey, and the effect was almost instantaneous—I began to pour with sweat. Afterwards, almost everything sorted itself out. The aches subsided, my temperature dropped, I could vomit, and I was soon in a deep, healing sleep. The next day, I was well again. What happened was that the ginger in the tea "resolved" the fever in a manner that was as dramatic as the effect of any modern medication. Only, unlike acetaminophen or aspirin, it did not simply take away the symptoms while leaving the disease still there. It actually precipitated healing and encouraged a fast, natural recovery. It was then that I decided to research ginger.

I now realize that ginger is one of the most remarkable of remedies. In the sophisticated world of Oriental medicine, it ranks as one of the best. A computerized study of all the constituents of thousands of Oriental remedies, carried out by Professor Izrael Brekhman's team from the Far East Science Centre of the former Soviet Union, showed that ginger was the fifth most frequently used of all Oriental remedies. Its role is unique; no other herb or spice can be substituted. What it does, according to Oriental medicine, is to "carry" other remedies into the body by aiding their absorption and distribution through the bloodstream and into the organs. The Chinese also use it to aid the flow of energy, immunity, and fluids throughout the body and to wake up tired organs. Science confirms that it opens the blood vessels, creates sweating and warmth, stimulates the heart, and thins the blood.

Ginger has some unique effects on the intestines. It is the only herb or spice we know that can prevent motion sickness, and it is the best known remedy for nausea. A clinical study conducted at St. Bartholomew's Hospital in London demonstrated that ginger is more effective than conventional anti-emetic drugs at preventing the very unpleasant nausea and vomiting that often occur when patients wake up from anesthesia after surgery. It is helpful to the digestive system in many other ways, too.

Ginger's effects on fever are also rather special. Ginger is the only remedy that most people have on hand to treat such a common occurrence as a viral fever. And, as already mentioned, no competing remedies exist for most of these uses of ginger, either in modern medicine's armory or in the herbal medicine chest. Besides being unique, ginger—like all medicinal foods—is inexpensive, easy to prepare, extremely safe, and readily available.

You now have some idea of ginger's value, and you will learn more in the following chapters. In addition, you will learn about ginger as part of our heritage, as part of our culture, and as part of our diet. A wealth of interesting information exists.

Ginger has entered our language. We say that we want to "ginger up" somebody or something. The word "ginger" has come to mean a kind of mild, revitalizing stimulation that lies somewhere between the full-blown irritation of chili pepper and the refreshing arousal of a cold shower or a cup of coffee. Most of us need to ginger up our bodies and our minds. In the following chapters, we will learn how to do so.

CHAPTER 2

Ginger and the Circulatory System

Ginger is a warm and pungent remedy. We have only to bite into it, to feel its taste and aromatic warmth spreading through us, to realize that it may be able to warm up some sluggish body processes and get them moving. This implies that it can treat health problems associated with cooling down, slowing down, or inactivity. The most important such health problem is heart disease. To know why ginger can do this, and to understand whether we really need to stoke our inner fires with ginger, we need to look more closely at our society's chief health problem and at how it arises from our lifestyle and environment.

CAUSES OF POOR CIRCULATION

Heart disease is the main cause of death and disability in the modern world. Some two-thirds of the Western population have elevated blood cholesterol levels, and around half will have a heart attack, stroke, or other circulation-based problem listed on their death certificates. The source of all this circulatory sickness is not simple to identify precisely, since circulatory problems are caused by many aspects of our lifestyle. We know, however, that primitive people do not suffer from these problems when they remain in their natural environments but they do when they migrate to towns. Moreover, when animals are put into a modern human environment, they too fall prey to the same kinds of heart and circulatory diseases.

We also know, after an immense research effort, that certain factors in our lifestyle increase the risks. Smoking is an obvious one. Another is lack of exercise, and another still is inherited susceptibility to heart attack or raised blood cholesterol. Fatty diets and a lot of cholesterol floating about in the circulatory system act together to increase risk, but this also is not the whole story; we know that people can eat fatty diets, as they did in our grandparents' day, without being the worse for it. Indeed, research done on groups like the Bedouin of Israel and Egypt shows that when people live amid nature, they eat mostly meat but have a low level of heart disease; whereas when they move into cities and civilization, they begin to suffer from heart disease, even though their diets become much more vegetarian. From this kind of evidence, and from looking at personality and behavior, the idea has arisen that stress greatly increases the risk of circulatory diseases. Stress is hard to define precisely, but in general it is associated with living in a state of too much arousal and nonspecific psychological imbalance, with a lack of inner peace and well-being.

All this, however, is well known today, so let us now go a little deeper in our examination. All the influences just mentioned tend to interact with one another. For example, stress raises blood cholesterol levels as least as much as a fatty diet does. Elevated blood cholesterol encourages the formation of fatty deposits that coat the arteries with plaque. Plaque-coated arteries (atherosclerosis) reduce organ function and lead to high blood pressure, which strains the heart. And so on. All these influences tend to produce similar internal changes, of which a heart attack is the end result. The arteries gradually become blocked by the fatty deposits, which causes blood flow to become restricted, which raises blood pressure. The flow of blood and body fluids to the limbs and surface of the body is reduced, leading to coldness, lessened sweating, and reduced elimination. The tissues get less blood and oxygen, which leads to more tiredness and poorer functioning by many of the body's organs, including (and especially) the heart.

We can look at all the causes of poor circulation to find the similarities between them. Smoking, for example, causes harm by constricting the blood vessels, not only in the lungs but all through the body. Lack of exercise causes the blood vessels to lose flexibility, making them similar to rusty floodgates that fail to allow sufficient blood to flow through. As the body is more and more underused, the flow stagnates more and more. The same happens from ingesting too much food and living with too much stress. All these factors lead to the blood vessels becoming closed, crusty, or inflexible. Indeed, one element of atherosclerosis is calcium deposits exactly like those inside a kettle. There cannot be a stronger indication than this of the nature of the problem.

In traditional medicine, this whole process is described as a "cooling off," or "slowing down." Even in modern medicine, we talk about circulatory disease as a "degenerative" disease, or a disease of "atrophy," meaning wasting away. We talk about "hardening of the arteries." Whereas in modern medicine the problem is looked at descriptively, or anatomically, in traditional medicine it is regarded as a process. The hardening of the arteries is just an end result of the slowing down of the flow of the metabolism, the flow of life energy, which allows plaque to be deposited like junk in a slow-moving stream. In traditional medicine, the treatment is to warm up the system, to get it moving again. For example, one classic remedy for circulation problems is garlic. Garlic is pungent and warming. It reduces cholesterol and thins the blood, helping to keep the arteries open. Another classic remedy is ginkgo, which works by expanding and relaxing the blood vessels on the surface of the body. Exercise is now known to be perhaps the best method to get the circulation moving and to open the blood vessels, especially the vast network of vessels that supplies the muscles and periphery of the body. Relaxation techniques and meditation reduce stress internally and relax not only the blood vessels but the entire body. Relaxation warms up the periphery, especially the hands and feet, as the blood vessels expand.

HEATING FROM WITHIN

Ginger certainly can make you sweat! This is a common experience among people who consume it. The warmth that ginger brings to the body is the basis for its action on the circulatory system. Imagine a hot bath or sauna. The heat spreads through the body, opening the channels; relaxing the tightness in the muscles, including those that constrict the blood vessels; and spreading the body's fluids evenly throughout the tissues, including in the outer areas of the body, which are most often deprived. Ginger works like a sauna, but from the inside out rather than from the outside in.

Cayenne pepper also works this way and is a constituent of many of the herbalist's professional preparations for the treatment of circulatory disease. Ginger is like cayenne, but it is milder, less irritating, and more suitable for self-treatment. It is also the preferred warming remedy in Oriental herbalism.

GINGER IN ORIENTAL MEDICINE

Oriental medicine understands ginger, one of its fundamental remedies, very well. It classifies ginger according to the way it is prepared. The classifications include:

- *Dried ginger.* Dried ginger is regarded as the hottest, most pungent, and spiciest type of ginger. It is used to warm the middle of the body and to stimulate the *yang Qi*, which is the basic vitality and body warmth. It disperses blockages that are hampering the blood, energy, digestion, metabolism, or body fluids. In other words, it really gets things moving. It is used for cold hands and feet, chills, weakness, poor digestion and vomiting, and weak circulation.

  Since ginger acts primarily on the stomach, lung, and spleen *meridians*, or energy paths, it is very useful for driving out colds, mucus, coughs, and bronchial infections (see Chapter 4). The Chinese use it when the weather or climate is cold and damp, to prevent chills, rheumatic conditions, and similar afflictions.

  The *Shang han lun*, a classical Chinese text, says: "Thus ginger has a stimulating action on the internal organs, with a warming effect besides. It adjusts the metabolism, eliminates excess fluids that have become stagnant in the body, dispels gas and aids digestion. The remedy is helpful in releasing obstruction and distention beneath the heart [in the digestive system]."

- *Fresh ginger.* Fresh ginger is spicy, warm, and aromatic.

It concentrates its action on the surface of the body to induce sweating, release toxins, and improve circulation in the skin and limbs. The Chinese use it especially for fevers and chills, aches and pains, acute rheumatic conditions, coughs, headaches, and some skin problems. Fresh ginger is most like the sauna described on page 16; it can be called sweat therapy. It is used preventively when the skin is cold and the circulation is poor. It is also used occasionally like dried ginger for colds and rheumatic conditions arising from the winter season or cold weather.

- *Roasted or baked ginger.* Roasted or baked ginger is relevant only in Oriental medicine. It is dried ginger that, after being baked, has lost its pungency and is bitter and warm. It does not disperse blockages or open blood vessels or body-fluid channels. Instead, it helps the spleen make and hold blood in its vessels, a process that the Chinese quaintly describe as "rallying the blood." It is used for intestinal bleeding, gynecological problems, and recovery from injury.

In Oriental medicine, ginger is never used on its own. Instead, it is always used in combination with other herbs and spices. Oriental doctors make a diagnosis based on bodily signs, read with great sensitivity. The surface signs—particularly the strength and steadiness of the pulses, color and texture of the tongue and skin, tenderness, and distribution of warmth over the body—are all indications of how well the functions inside the body are being performed. Remedies are designed to adjust these functions. For example, a weak and hollow pulse that does not bounce back properly when pressed is a sign of a hardened or cholesterol-blocked blood vessel. An Oriental doctor will prepare a mixture to stimulate the heart using herbs such as Chinese aconite, Chinese sage, ginger, licorice, poria, and Chinese angelica, or Tang kuei. The exact mixture would depend on the constitution of the patient and the imbalances in his or her various body systems. For example, Tang kuei would be used if there were a lack of nutrition and oxygen in the blood, leading to pain upon exercise; poria would be used if edema (fluid retention) were a symptom; aconite, if the heart required a boost. Ginger is an assistant to all these herbs and spices because it carries them—or "conducts" them, as the Chinese say—to the place where they need to work. Ginger is almost always needed to get the circulation moving.

SCIENTIFIC SUPPORT FOR GINGER'S CARDIOVASCULAR EFFECTS

As is true for many herbs and spices, there has been little investment in clinical studies on ginger's classical uses by people. There have been no clinical studies at all on ginger's effects on the circulation. However, there have been a number of laboratory studies using animals, and these confirm the traditional picture just described.

Small amounts of ginger extract injected into animals caused the animals' heart muscles to beat more strongly. Studies at the Pharmacy Department of Tokushima-Bunri University, Tokushima, Japan, demonstrated that the pungent components of ginger are able to stimulate the major heart muscle to beat with more contractile force. The heart actually beats more slowly and more strongly. In addition, studies at several other Japanese research centers and universities have confirmed that when ginger extract or its active ingredients are given to animals, blood pressure is lowered by ten to fifteen points for up to several hours. This is a significant reduction.

Little is known about how ginger actually achieves this. Very few scientists have been curious enough to investigate where the plant's little molecules end up in the body. One clue was located by, again, Japanese scientists, this time at the University of Kyoto. These scientists found that pungent molecules from both ginger and cayenne pepper make a beeline for the adrenal glands. There, the molecules stimulate the adrenal medullae, the central segments of these hormone-producing glands, to produce their messengers, one of which is adrenaline. Adrenaline stimulates the circulation and warms the body. However, it must be stressed that this can be only a small part of the picture, since adrenaline does other things that ginger certainly does not do, such as stimulating alertness and constricting circulation in the stomach and in the interior of the body. Constricting circulation is certainly the opposite of what ginger does.

What these studies tell us is that ginger relaxes and opens the blood vessels in the periphery of the body and lets more blood and body fluids through. Because the vessels are open, the heart does not have to pump as hard to overcome resistance; it is easier for the heart to send the blood coursing along. This lowers the blood pressure. Ginger also seems to gently stimulate the heart because the heart contracts more strongly. And since the heart does not need to work as hard, the heart rate, or speed of pumping, slows down. In other words, the evidence indicates that, as the Chinese say, ginger spreads the fluids more easily around the body, thus taking the load off the heart, which can then slow down and ease the blood pressure.

Another helpful effect of ginger is that it lowers cholesterol levels in the liver and the blood. Studies by Dr. S. Gujral and colleagues at the University of Baroda, Gujarat, India, have shown that if animals are fed a cholesterol-loaded diet, with foods such as slabs of butter on concessionary pieces of bread, the cholesterol level in the blood rises dramatically. Ginger was shown to be capable of preventing much of this rise, provided it is taken over a period of time; it does not work immediately.

Other researchers have confirmed this observation. They have found that as soon as ginger is added to a cholesterol-rich meal fed to an animal, cholesterol is excreted from the body before it reaches the blood vessels. These researchers suggested that ginger works in the same way as a variety of resins from plants and other herbs and spices—by removing cholesterol from the body via the liver and digestive system. However, ginger's action in this area is not as strong and specific as, for example, that of garlic.

GINGER AND BLOOD-CLOTTING

The other side of the coin regarding ginger's ability to free the circulation is its action on blood-clotting factors. This action has been intensively studied, especially at the Institute of Community Health of the University of Odense, Denmark. There, Dr. K. Srivastava has been investigating the cell fragments called platelets that are involved in the first stage in the blood-clotting process. Platelets stick to wound edges and initiate clots that lead to healing, but they can also stick to the plaque on the insides of narrowed arteries and produce unwanted clots there. Such clots can precipitate coronary thrombosis (a heart attack) or cerebrovascular accident (stroke). These kinds of clots are extreme cases. But microclots can also occur, restricting circulation. People with circulatory problems usually have blood that clots too easily, which is why doctors often prescribe small amounts of aspirin to reduce clotting.

Japanese scientists are currently testing an anti-clotting remedy to compete with aspirin. The remedy consists very simply of capsules containing sixty milligrams of one of ginger's main medicinal components, a substance called shogaol. The remedy is not yet available.

The Danish team from Odense found that ginger is a very powerful inhibitor of the clumping of platelets, the very first stage in the clotting process. Ginger was clearly found to make the blood less sticky. But the researchers were able to go one step further. They were able to look at the mechanism of the process, and they found something very interesting—the platelets were less sticky because they made less of substances called thromboxane and prostaglandins. These are local chemical messengers that have been greatly researched recently as the agents of pain, inflammation, fever, and other body-defense reactions. It is clear that many remedies that treat body-defense reactions work by limiting the local messengers. Aspirin, for example, has a very similar effect, both on the platelets and on the local messengers.

This knowledge can help us to understand the way ginger works and to put it in perspective as a remedy. Several medicinal foods are known to reduce prostaglandins and thromboxane, but they do so in ways that are different and too complex to describe here. For example, garlic, like ginger, reduces blood stickiness, but since it does not have the same kind of effect on prostaglandins as ginger or cloves do, it does not reduce fever and pain as they do. We do not know for certain whether ginger's ability to open blood vessels and warm the body is also connected with prostaglandins, but it would come as no surprise if it were. This is because expansion and contraction of blood vessels, as well as local heating, are among the functions of the prostaglandins and of similar chemicals.

TAKING GINGER FOR THE CIRCULATION

If we regard ginger as a kind of internal sauna, we will not be far off the mark. Ginger should be taken regularly by people whose circulation needs awakening and warming. This includes people who:

- Suffer from atherosclerosis and are at risk for heart disease due to poor diet, lack of exercise, or a similar reason.

- Smoke heavily.

- Have cold hands or feet.

- Feel cold or lack vitality and energy, especially during cold weather.

- Have "poor circulation"—that is, inadequate blood supply to the skin and periphery of the body, manifesting as slow wound healing and muscle pain upon exercise.

As the Chinese say, ginger is only one weapon in a campaign to restore healthy circulation. It should be combined with other medicinal foods and treatments. The exact mixture will depend on the individual, and for this reason, a sincere attempt to prevent or reduce a circulatory problem should include professional assistance in designing a personalized, or customized, herbal and lifestyle regime.

Ginger combines very well with other methods for improving general health and the circulation. In particular, it goes well with herbs like hawthorn, mistletoe, and lily of the valley, which reduce blood pressure and strengthen the heart, because ginger, unlike these other herbs, spreads body fluids throughout the body. It helps herbs and spices that relax the heart and reduce stress and nervous stimulation, such as Chinese seneca, or milkwort, and Chinese dates, or jujube. It also goes well with garlic. Though ginger and garlic are similar in some ways—both are pungent, lower cholesterol, and reduce blood stickiness—garlic is far more effective at reducing cholesterol and body fat and at dissolving blood clots. Ginger is more effective at improving circulation and strengthening the heart. Therefore, ginger and garlic accentuate as well as complement each other.

Ginger is obviously an excellent companion to dietary measures. It is particularly useful during a mild fast or change of diet. It helps to stimulate energy and circulation and also helps to eliminate toxins, promote sweating, and clean the body. It is simple to add to the diet. It is also a useful companion to an exercise program, since it encourages sweating and the elimination of wastes. However, it should not be taken by individuals who overheat easily or get very red and sweaty.

People in cold climates often become constricted, in body and sometimes in spirit. If these people also suffer from the ills of modern life, their circulation is assailed from two directions. Perhaps this is why circulatory problems seem so intractable among North Americans and northern Europeans, while the Mexicans, Italians, and French seem to get off very lightly despite an equal dose of unhealthy food, cigarettes, and other negative factors. This points to the special value of ginger for those in northern climes. It is clear that we have heeded the message in relation to garlic, which has returned to our lives in a big way in recent years. Now it is time to add ginger.

CHAPTER 3

Ginger and the Digestive System

The most important and best known use of ginger is for the digestive system. Ginger is the classic medicine for fighting nausea, vomiting, poor digestion, and indigestion; for protecting against stomach ulcers; and for assisting the absorption of foods and medications into the body. Before we examine these uses in more detail, we will take a look at the digestive system itself.

TUMMY TROUBLES

Dr. Johnson, the acerbic eighteenth-century British author, joked, "He who does not mind his belly will hardly mind anything else." But having an upset stomach is part of daily life for many people. It is regarded as so normal that people look at you in astonishment if you say that you never have such a problem. Indeed, the term "to belly-ache" has entered our language as a slang expression meaning "to grumble."

The digestive system is intimately connected to the rest of the body, as well as to the mind. At the same time, it can be said to have a kind of intelligence of its own. If you could look into the stomach, you would see there the reflections of thoughts passing through the mind. Where do you feel embarrassment, stage fright, and anxiety? Certainly not in the brain, where these emotions arise. The Japanese recognize this to an extent—their word for generosity, or "largeness of personality," translates as "large belly." The movements, rumbles, redness, squirts of digestive juices, drips of acid, activity of millions of little "fingers" (called villi) that take in fat droplets, control of events by a complex network of local and long-distance hormones, and even the work of an entire immune system are all there in the digestive system, taking part as the digestion busily responds to all the changes in the body, in the mind, in the emotions, and in the environment.

For this reason, we can no longer look at the stomach as being simply a kind of flask full of juices that breaks down everything that comes its way. This "urn and churn" model is out of date. Consider some common stomach problems. Indigestion occurs when the intestine is given too much to handle. Some people have systems that can handle more than others, and some have systems that are extremely sensitive to even very small amounts of certain foods. Gas and colic are the result of eating too much of the wrong kind of food, such as beans or cow's milk, both of which have types of sugar that are inadequately digested. Undigested sugars are prey for intestinal bacteria, which produce gas and toxins as they devour the sugars. Non-food causes of indigestion include stress and anxiety, which can wreak havoc immediately.

Nausea and vomiting are normal, common reactions to poisons, alcohol, infections, dizziness, rocking movements, fetal waste products (during pregnancy), and shocks (such as the sight of blood). In all these cases, nausea and vomiting are the body's attempt to purify itself naturally. A gastric ulcer is an open area where the stomach has tried to digest itself due to long-term anxiety and stress. It occurs because the constant alarm reaction not only restricts the blood supply to the stomach but also changes the hormonal environment there. According to naturopaths, allergies and even some rheumatic problems are the result of harmful and undigested substances being let into the body because of inadequate digestion. Such problems are clearly mind-body problems.

Traditional medicine, especially Oriental medicine, describes how the environment, the constitution, and individual behavior affect the quality of the digestive process. For example, if digestive vital power (*Qi*) is lacking due to overwork, symptoms such as abdominal pain and distension, lethargy, and indigestion can result; the individual lacks sufficient power to move food smartly down the digestive conveyor belt. If cold has invaded the system, even from a change in the weather, the result could be abdominal pain and poor digestion, leading to a build-up of toxins in the body, headaches, and similar symptoms. The proper digestive "fire" to burn, or transform, food into body energy, power, and health is a key concept of traditional medicine.

GINGER IN AYURVEDIC MEDICINE

The most intricate understanding of the process of digestion comes from Indian traditional medicine, Ayurveda. Ayurveda is an extremely sophisticated system that, like Oriental medicine, has its own theories of life, of matter, and of health and disease. These theories are part of Indian culture, philosophy, and spiritual beliefs.

Ayurveda sees our universe as composed of five basic *elements—earth, air, fire, water,* and *space.* According to Ayurveda, the West received this teaching from the East through Pythagoras and the early Greeks. The five basic elements are codes for qualities. *Earth,* for example, means solidity, passivity, and materiality. *Fire* is energy, transformation, and heat. *Water* is cohesiveness, attraction, and dampness. *Air* represents life, movement, and action. *Space* is the background against which the other four elements exist.

The body is composed of its own qualities, called *humors—Vata,* which corresponds best to the air element within ether; *Pitta,* which is largely the biological fire element located within water; and *Kapha,* which is the water element, with a base in earth. These three humors, or *doshas,* govern different body types, which are susceptible to ailments resulting from an imbalance of the dosha. The body types and the ailments to which they are prone are:

- *Vata type.* This body type tends to be tall, thin, and bony, with dry, cool skin. These people generally are erratic in their habits, adaptable, indecisive, nervous, and sensitive. They talk fast, sleep lightly, and generally do not sweat. They lean toward air-type illnesses, including nervous-system problems, arthritic and rheumatic complaints, and all kinds of pains. Stomach problems, such as diarrhea, usually involve gas, bloating, pain, little urination, and inadequate digestive function.

  Ginger, according to Ayurveda, is good for Vata-type digestive problems, since it helps absorption and digestive functions, warms the intestines, and treats cramps, gas, and colicky pain.

- *Pitta type.* This body type tends to be medium in build and muscular, with warm, rosy skin and soft hair. Pitta-type people are marked by moderate speech, a strong appetite, and loose motions. They sweat more than normal, sleep soundly, and are critical, argumentative, and prone to anger. The ailments that tend to affect them include inflammations, infections, liver problems, ulcers, and skin rashes. Any digestive problems are likely to be more "fiery"—that is, of the diarrhea type—than the digestive problems of Vata- and Kapha-type individuals. Diarrhea in a Pitta-type person generally looks like bacterial dysentery. It is hot, accompanied by fever and thirst, and involves frequent passing of thin liquid.

Pitta people do not do well with ginger and, for the most part, do not need it because they are by nature fiery enough. In fact, some of their problems are the result of their being too fiery. Instead of ginger, Ayurveda recommends a less astringent, more soothing remedy for the digestion, such as coriander, cumin, caraway, or fennel.

- *Kapha type.* This body type leans toward being heavier, stouter, and slower than the other two, with a pale complexion, oily hair, and thick skin. These are people of constant habits, with a moderate digestion and a tendency to have mucus. They are likely to be calm and sentimental, and are sometimes dull. They speak slowly and sleep deeply. The illnesses that affect them include bronchial problems, edema, mucus problems, swollen glands, growths, stomach problems, and ear, nose, and throat problems. A digestive complaint like diarrhea is accompanied by heaviness, lethargy, and weakness, with the passing of a great deal of mucus.

According to Ayurveda, ginger is particularly good for Kapha types. Consumed as part of the diet, it helps to absorb and balance watery or oily foods, and it prevents the heaviness and obesity that can result from eating such foods. Ginger helps counterbalance too much sugar, too much dairy, too much alcohol, too much fruit, and too much meat. It does this better than pepper or mustard, which, though pungent, can be too drying. In general, ginger is good for Kapha types to counteract a tendency toward lethargy, congestion, and stagnation.

An important concept in Ayurveda is that of *Agni*, or digestive and metabolic fire. If food and other inputs are properly burned, processed, and digested, they will not create toxins, called *Ama*, which collect in deposits around the body. The cholesterol that clogs the arteries is a kind of Ama deposit. Arthritic deterioration of the joints is also an Ama problem.

Ayurveda employs herbs and spices, oils, yoga, massage, dietary principles, colors, gems, minerals, and almost anything imaginable as a therapeutic tool. One of the many Ayurveda principles that should help us understand ginger better is that of the six *tastes*. Like Oriental medicine, Ayurveda classifies herbs and spices by taste. The six tastes are:

1. *Sweet* (for example, angelica, licorice, lovage, and fruit such as dates or figs), which tends to soothe, harmonize, stimulate the bowels, nourish, and support the body's immune system.

2. *Salty* (for example, seaweed), which mildly sedates, regulates body fluids, relaxes tissues, stimulates the digestion in small amounts, and purges the bowels in larger amounts.

3. *Sour* (for example, cider vinegar, lemon, tamarind, and yogurt), which tends to stimulate, calm the stomach, relieve thirst, and nourish.

4. *Pungent* (for example, ginger, cayenne, and garlic), which stimulates, improves the functioning of body systems, causes sweating, removes extra liquid from

the body, and promotes heat, digestion, and metabolism.

5. *Bitter* (for example, aloe, feverfew, seneca, and wormwood), which cleanses, detoxifies, reduces inflammation, and stimulates elimination, immunity, and secretions.

6. *Astringent* (for example, plantain, raspberry leaf, and yarrow), which stops bleeding, heals wounds, reduces liquids in the body, and prevents diarrhea.

Ayurvedic medicine considers ginger a pungent spice par excellence. Ginger does not have the concentrated irritant pungency of cayenne or chili, which can sometimes be too strong. Yet it is irritant enough to challenge the muscles and the blood vessels and to wake them up. It also challenges the internal organs, particularly the digestive system, in which it is said to awaken the Agni. Symptoms of low Agni include poor digestion, poor absorption, poor circulation, gas, constipation, poor resistance, a tendency to colds and influenza, congestion, body odor, and obesity. (Obesity is a problem because the body does not have sufficient fire to balance the water.) All of these problems are precisely those that ginger treats.

When Agni is improved, Ama is destroyed. Poisons and undigested wastes are removed. Digestive symptoms such as nausea that are the result of toxins are treated. And in the long term, the build-up of toxins that produces conditions such as atherosclerosis, allergies, and rheumatic problems is prevented.

The basic concepts just discussed lead to some interesting conclusions about how we may be able to use ginger. For example, if we fast, we would be well advised to take ginger tea, especially with lemon, to maintain our metabolic fire. We would be less tired, and detoxification would be more complete. If we take a laxative, we might find it too strong, causing cramps and gas. By taking ginger with it, we could preserve our Agni, preventing such symptoms. Indeed, any medication we take can have a negative effect on the digestion as it passes through the system. Ginger can protect the stomach against damage, which is another reason it is so frequently an ingredient in herbal mixtures.

WESTERN HERBALISM

Western herbalists have a remarkably similar attitude toward ginger, although their language is rather different. They describe ginger as a "stimulating carminative." A *carminative* is an herb or spice that calms and supports the digestive system. It soothes the stomach, relieves gas, eases cramps, and generally encourages normal digestion and absorption. The carminative herbs and spices all contain aromatic oils. Examples include the mint family, melissa, caraway, fennel, cinnamon, ginger, and chamomile. Others are verbena, which is the French after-dinner tisane, and aniseed, which no restaurant in India, even the simplest roadside stall, would fail to give a customer after a meal.

According to the Western view, carminative herbs and spices work mainly by relaxing the smooth muscles that make the digestive system function. They also relax the small muscles around the blood vessels of the stomach, allowing more blood into the stomach and improving the organ's functioning. Some early European research involved the use of a gastroscope to examine the stomach while carminatives were taken. As soon as the herbs entered it, the stomach, as seen through the gastroscope, became redder and more folded. This demonstrated that the herbs improved the blood circulation. Improved blood circulation, along with relaxed muscles, prevents cramping and pain. It moves gas along and speeds up digestion. Spicing our food with carminative herbs obviously makes excellent sense.

All the carminatives do not work in exactly the same way, however. For example, the mint family is warming and relaxes the muscles well, so it is especially effective against stomach cramps. Chamomile has an additional cleansing action against bacteria, so it is effective against stomach upset. The umbelliferous seeds—aniseed, cumin, fennel, and caraway—are not very warming but improve digestion, especially the secretion of digestive juices. Therefore, they are especially effective against gas and in "oiling the wheels of the digestive machinery." Ginger is particularly good at opening blood vessels and at stimulating absorption and circulation. Because of this, it is classed as a stimulating carminative (unlike fennel, caraway, and chamomile, which are relaxing carminatives).

This Western view of ginger fits well not only with the Ayurvedic concept but also with the Oriental view, which similarly describes ginger as warming to the center and able to improve the digestive fires. In Oriental medicine, ginger is said to disperse blockages. Food, blood, fluids, and energy are all stimulated to move along more smartly. Vomiting, nausea, indigestion, gas, and stomach pains are seen by Oriental doctors to be the result of "cold," or "congested," or "weak" digestive functioning. Ginger has the effect of warming up the digestive system, helping it to complete all its physiological actions.

Oriental and Ayurvedic medicine regard an ailment such as dysentery as a problem of weak digestion rather than as an infection, which is how Western medicine sees it. An Oriental or Ayurvedic physician would ask, How would the bacteria survive if digestion proceeded at a normal pace?

Infection can occur only in a stagnant pool, not in a free-flow-ing stream. Consequently, an Oriental or Ayurvedic physi-cian would include ginger in a mixture to cure bacterial dysentery. In one clinical study, a hospital in Shandong, China, reported that about ten grams a day of a paste of raw ginger and brown sugar was used to treat fifty patients with bacterial dysentery. About 70 percent of the patients were cured in under five days. The rest took a little longer.

NAUSEA, VOMITING, AND MOTION SICKNESS

In the autumn of 1985, eighty healthy naval cadets boarded the Danish training ship Danmark, a fully rigged but smallish sailing vessel, and sailed off to the rough waters of the Skagerrak, an arm of the North Sea in Scandinavia. There, these inexperienced sailors met swells of three to five yards and, not surprisingly, two-thirds of the men became ill. The ship's doctor handed out pills and assessed the severity of the well-known symptoms—nausea, dizzi-ness, vomiting, and cold sweating. The cadets had no notion of what was inside the pills, and they might have been surprised. Forty of them received pills containing only sugar—that is, placebos, or pretend pills. The other forty were given pills containing ground ginger root. When the director of the study, Dr. Aksel Gronved of the Svendborg Hospital, statistically analyzed the results, he found that the cadets who took the ginger pills fared much better. In some cases, the symptoms were halved, and the effect lasted for at least four hours.

Dried ginger is not only effective against motion sick-ness but also appears to be better than the usual drug, Dramamine. In a study at Brigham Young University in Provo, Utah, thirty-six students went through the ex-tremely uncomfortable process of sitting in a chair that revolved while also rising and falling. In addition, the students were blindfolded and told to keep their heads tilted to one side. Twelve of the students were given capsules of Dramamine, twelve were given an inert placebo, and the remaining twelve were given just under one gram of dried ginger. They did not know who received what or even what the study was examining. All their symptoms were recorded. None of the students who took the placebo was able to stay in the chair for the full period of six minutes. All the placebo recipients were very sick, and by three minutes, their symptoms were rated at around 900 on a subjective scale. The Dramamine recipients fared a little better. By four minutes, their symptoms were up to a score of only around 550, but they, too, could not stay in the chair for the full time. Only the students in the ginger group lasted the full course; and by six minutes, their symptom score was only about 200.

Several similar studies have been conducted and have put ginger in the public eye as the only serious natural remedy for motion sickness. In particular, the pioneering work of American herbal researcher Dr. Daniel Mowrey has awakened public interest in this use of ginger. In 1982, Dr. Mowrey published a report in the prestigious British medical journal *Lancet* that showed that volunteers taking ginger were much less likely to suffer motion sickness in a laboratory "rotating chair" simulator than volunteers not taking ginger. It is well known that the conventional medications for motion sickness, such as Dramamine, work on the nervous centers in the brain that cause the upset and therefore may induce drowsiness and lethargy. Because of this, these medications cannot be used by automobile drivers, sailors, or astronauts—the very people who need them the most.

Ginger is widely used in the East for motion sickness. More than one traveler from China has recounted how the bus seemed to reek of it as people chewed their way through small pieces from time to time. The best dose is one gram of dried ginger, taken at least a half-hour before traveling.

Nausea and vomiting can have a variety of causes. Are there cases where ginger should not be used? Yes. Occasionally, vomiting should be encouraged rather than suppressed. If poison or bad food is the cause of the nausea, vomiting is useful and can be stimulated by the herb lobelia or by a teaspoonful of salt in a glass of water. In cases of nausea that have nervous origins, ginger can be used but should be accompanied by relaxation techniques, warming of the body, sleep, and perhaps a mint or chamomile tea. When there is hyperacidity, gastric ulcers, or lack of digestive juices, both Indian and Western medicine prefer the use of aromatic bitter herbs, not ginger, to stimulate the secretion of digestive fluids. These herbs include gentian, aloe, marshmallow, boldo (a Chilean evergreen shrub), and angelica.

MORNING SICKNESS AND DRUG SIDE EFFECTS

For most cases of nausea and vomiting, ginger is useful because it acts on the stomach itself as an energizing balm, rather than on the brain centers as a depressant, the way modern antinausea drugs do. Therefore, the precise cause of the ill feeling is not so relevant—ginger can help to prevent nausea stemming from a variety of causes. For example, ginger in tea, capsule, or tablet form is perhaps the most effective remedy available for morning sickness during pregnancy. A clinical trial involving thirty women with the most severe kind of morning sickness, *hyperemesis gravidarum*, was reported in the *European Journal of Obstetrics and Gynaecology* in 1991. It showed that one gram of ground ginger per day greatly reduced the symptoms and in some cases eliminated them.

Remember, however, that the fewer remedies that are taken during pregnancy, the better. Herbs and spices taken in large amounts rank as medicines, and therefore should not be consumed unnecessarily during this time. Avoid excessive doses. Also remember that morning sickness is not an inevitable and necessary curse. It is the result of imbalances within the system that allow accumulation of toxins from the fetus. The body becomes overloaded with waste products and tries to remove them by vomiting. Natural therapists and herbalists often recommend nutritional support to improve the condition of the blood. For example, alfalfa, nettle, oats, kelp, pollen, spirulina (a nutritive alga), and vitamin B complex can be of help.

Nausea and vomiting may also occur as side effects of medications, anesthetics, or other toxins in the body. Ginger is highly effective in such cases. This was well illustrated in the study mentioned in Chapter 1 in which sixty patients at St. Bartholomew's Hospital were given ginger to fight postoperative nausea and vomiting. Nausea and vomiting are side effects of the anesthetic used during surgery and are particularly unpleasant and difficult to handle. Doctors are reluctant to give additional medications, since these medications may cause drowsiness. Only half a gram of ginger was given before surgery to a group of women undergoing major gynecological procedures. For comparison, another group was given ten milligrams of metoclopramide, a conventional antinausea drug. A third group received a placebo. Those taking the ginger had much less nausea and vomiting than did the others. None of the women taking the ginger needed an antivomiting drug after the operation, in contrast to those in the other groups. The authors, Dr. M. E. Bone and colleagues, pointed out that "there has been no real reduction during the last 50 years in [post]operative nausea and vomiting which remains at 30%, despite the continued introduction of new anti-emetics ... Ginger has the major advantage over other substances in that it does not have any recorded side-effects."

Not surprisingly, doctors in India, which has an indigenous medical system still intact, had already thought of this. A special ginger-containing remedy called Gasex is used in some hospitals after surgery to prevent nausea, gas, and other intestinal discomforts. Tests show Gasex to be highly effective.

Some very distressing consequences of taking anti-cancer drugs are the nausea and vomiting that are the usual side effects. Ginger helps reduce these symptoms, too, as supported by preliminary research. A clinical study of the use of ginger for nausea from chemotherapy was carried out in 1987 by Dr. J. C. Pace at the University of Alabama in Birmingham. Leukemia patients who took ginger tablets along with their chemotherapy reported less nausea than did those patients who took placebos.

CLEARING OUT POISONS

As mentioned earlier in this chapter, ginger, according to Ayurveda, increases Agni, or metabolic energy, and in so doing, reduces and destroys toxins in the body. In fact, since ginger opens blood vessels, spreads fluids properly throughout the body, stimulates the flow of bile and waste products from the liver, and causes sweating, it probably also helps to dump poisons and toxins out of the body. The longer toxins sit around in one place, the more harm they do. This is another case in which we can apply the well-worn image of the stagnant pool.

In traditional Oriental medicine, removing toxins is one of the major uses of ginger. Ginger is given as an antidote to poisoning from foods, drugs, or other herbs or spices. It is added to herbal mixtures as an antidote to the toxic ingredients in the mixture. This ability of ginger is recognized by physicians and herbalists in the West, too. Peter Holmes reminds us of this in his classic text *The Energetics of Western Herbs*. He quotes the British herbalist Henry Barham, who stated in 1794 that ginger is "a corrective of many medicines ... [which] taketh away their malice."

In modern China, ginger juice is used as an emergency remedy for poisoning. One teaspoon of juice is gargled and then swallowed, with another teaspoonful taken every four hours. Ginger juice presumably causes a great deal of sweating, heat, and stimulation, and is especially good against poisons that depress the body. In modern conventional medicine, stimulants, and even a slap in the face, are also given in such cases.

RESTORING PROPER DIGESTION

In Chapter 1, we discussed the reasons spices should be added to our food on a regular basis. Some of these reasons relate to the assistance that spices give our digestive system. Drawing largely from Ayurvedic knowledge, we will now look briefly at some other digestive problems.

Diarrhea has many causes, such as dysentery, bad food, nerves, viruses, and parasitic infestation. As we have seen, except in Pitta types, ginger—along with other spices, such as cardamom and coriander, and a bland, whole-grain diet—is used to promote absorption in the intestine. In addition, an astringent herb or spice, such as bilberry, cranesbill, tormentil, or garlic, may be used to stop infection and to dry inflammatory secretions.

In addition to having numerous causes, diarrhea also can be of several types, according to the Indian classification. Vata-type diarrhea can involve more pain, gas, and cramps, and not much liquid, while Kapha-type diarrhea tends to be cool, with more mucus. The above treatment is suitable for both. However, Pitta-type diarrhea, which is more watery, hot, and inflammatory, should not be treated with warming spices. Bitters such as gentian, wormwood, and goldenseal can instead be used.

Constipation is the mirror image of diarrhea, and it, too, can be the result of many factors, particularly a long-term diet with insufficient roughage and vegetables, insufficient physical activity, anxiety, overstimulation and overwork, medications, and other factors that slow the normal rhythms of the digestive system. Just as diarrhea does, constipation generates toxins that can cause long-term health problems, such as chronic headaches, as well as low immunity. This is now so well known that even the average family doctor will question patients about their bowel movements when investigating illness.

Generally, constipation is treated with a change in diet, which should begin with a fast that includes little except fruit and vegetable juices. Enemas, sweating therapy, and other detoxification procedures are helpful. Afterwards, a diet with plenty of roughage such as oatmeal, bran, and salad vegetables, as well as yogurt, whole grains, prunes, nuts, and cold-pressed oils, will often correct the problem.

Vata-type constipation is typically caused by lack of moisture in the digestive system. Symptoms include gas, bloating, pain, and headache. This type of constipation may be difficult to get rid of, but bulk laxatives such as psyllium or flax seed are often useful. Castor oil or olive oil may also be effective. If the constipation persists, a stronger laxative, such as rhubarb or senna, should be used. In all cases, ginger and other spices are very useful for keeping the digestive system functioning and also for counterbalancing the laxatives.

In Kapha-type, or water-type, constipation, the digestive system tends to be congested, with a lot of mucus or phlegm, which may also produce problems in the chest or throat. The afflicted individual feels lethargic and heavy and is generally overweight. Here, bulk laxatives, such as flax seed, should not be used, since they increase mucus. Bitter laxatives, such as aloe and senna, are effective, as are fasting and exercise. Again, ginger and hot, stimulating herbs such as pepper are effective.

Finally, the hot, Pitta-type constipation is often accompanied by fever, or is the result of fever, and may cause thirst, irritability, sweating, distention, and pain. For this kind of constipation, the best remedy is drinking a lot of liquids, eating a light diet of cooling raw foods, and taking a mild, bitter laxative, such as cascara, aloe, or yellow dock. Ginger and other hot spices are not recommended.

GINGER AND ABSORPTION

In the early part of the twentieth century, many health problems were considered to be the result of a disturbance in the normal intestinal flora, the rich culture of helpful bacteria in the intestine. At that time, spices were assumed to be of help because they were antibacterial, stopping invasions of the wrong bacteria. We now know that although this is correct—although the essential oils within spices are antibacterial as well as antioxidant and food-preserving—this is only a very small part of the picture. Thus, in the case of ginger, laboratory studies have demonstrated that ginger inhibits the bacteria in the colon that work away at undigested sugars, such as those from hard-to-digest beans. But ginger is also known now to have the more important action of encouraging more complete digestion and absorption of foods farther up in the digestive channel. This is better for preventing gas and digestive upsets than is the antibacterial action lower down.

The research into ginger's work in the digestive system is still very incomplete. Some evidence has been found that ginger, along with other spices, promotes secretion of digestive fluid. I have already mentioned that ginger can be seen to bring blood to the stomach walls and that it has been proven to be a cholagogue—that is, a medicine that stimulates the flow of bile—which is certainly an advantage in the digestion of fats and the elimination of wastes. Again, however, the studies that have shown this were done using animals and need to be confirmed by clinical work using humans before ginger can be expected to make its way back into pharmacopoeias.

One of the main reasons ginger is added to so many mixtures and prescriptions in Oriental and Indian traditional medicine is the way it helps the absorption of the other constituents. Ginger is often described as being the messenger or servant that brings other medicines to the sites at which they should act. In fact, some preliminary scientific evidence from India has shown that ginger can increase the absorption of pharmaceutical drugs and also protect the stomach from damage by aspirin and nonsteroidal anti-inflammatory drugs.

The potential use of ginger to normalize the digestion, as well as to help with the absorption of medications, herbs and spices, and nutrients, is fascinating. We would be able to reduce the dosage of a medicine or make it work more efficiently, thereby making it safer. Better nutrition would be the result if we combined our soups or our supplements with a little ginger, and our much-abused intestines would have a little protection from all the substances with which they have to cope.

Ginger itself is absorbed extremely fast. Research has shown that its pungent powerhouse molecules race into the body. In one second, they are through the stomach wall. No wonder they open the way for other substances to follow.

As we will see in Chapter 7, the famous folk rhyme on ginger seems to be very true: "Run, run, as fast as you can; you can't catch me, I'm the gingerbread man!"

CHAPTER 4

Ginger for Coughs, Colds, Aches, and Pains

L egend has it that King Henry VIII of England learned that ginger was good against the plague and recommended it to his subjects. Consequently, people began to eat gingerbread, baked in the shape of little men with round bellies. Whether this was to please the king or tease the king, or was a leftover of an ancient pagan rite, is anyone's guess. But this is the legendary origin of the gingerbread man.

In the early sixteenth century, with the plague threatening, eating ginger must have been rather like clutching at straws, for ginger is not an antibiotic, as we now know. However, it does have another, very useful function in the fight against colds, flu, viral infections, coughs, chronic bronchial problems, and low-grade infections of all kinds. As we have seen, it can warm the body, improve the circulation, and activate the body's defenses. This was even noted by modern medical practitioners, at least until recently, for ginger was described in pharmacopoeias as a cough and cold remedy, as well as a carminative and a flavoring agent.

Ginger does not attack viruses or bacteria specifically. Nor is it an expectorant—that is, a medicine that loosens mucous secretions, allowing a cough to get them out. Instead, it brings body fluids to affected areas, warming them up. This mobilizes the body's defenses, encouraging them to take the situation a little more seriously and not be so complacent and lethargic. As a result, in the case of a cough, secretions are increased, so phlegm becomes thinner and can be coughed up. Sweating is increased, driving out toxins or viruses. Immune-system functioning is increased, more white cells are produced, and, above all, circulation to all those hard-to-reach places is improved. Mustard plasters are a well-known folk remedy for bronchial problems. They are also heating and pungent, working in much the same way as ginger.

COLDS AND COUGHS

Colds, chills, coughs, bronchitis, flu, and catarrh (inflammation of the mucous membranes, especially in the nose and throat) are all signs of what the Chinese call "invading cold," or "invading damp." Cold and dampness have gotten into the system from the climate or environment and need to be driven out with warm, pungent remedies that encourage sweating. In these cases, Oriental medicine adds one more description—that these ailments are "exterior" conditions, disturbances of the outer areas of the body, not of its deep center, among the organs. For these conditions, we want ginger to work more on the exterior, producing sweating and improving peripheral circulation. As we saw in Chapter 2, fresh ginger is good at warming the exterior and provoking sweating. The fresh form of ginger is therefore better for colds, coughs, and respiratory problems.

There are many choices in the treatment of colds. In the

early stages, drink ginger tea with lemon and cloves or take ginger tablets. Vitamin C has been proven very helpful in nipping viral diseases, including colds, in the bud and greatly reducing their severity. Eat very lightly or not at all, and if you do eat, stay far away from oils, fats, and dairy products, all of which increase mucus and congestion (or Kapha, or phlegm). Once the cold is established, your focus should switch to clearing out the mucus and congestion and warming the inside of the body. Inhale sage tea or mentholated balm (a little balm in a bowl with steaming water). You can also put a tiny amount of balm on the nostril entrances to help clear the congestion. If you have a headache or sinus problem, massage the balm into your forehead and temples. Sage is a very effective herb for drying secretions and is our standby in these cases. Garlic and onions with honey is another helpful mixture. Continue taking ginger throughout your cold to keep up the sweating and the inner warmth. This can mean the difference between a cold that seems to drag on and one that is quickly overcome. Other herbs useful for colds are lemon balm and catnip. They all warm the body gently and help relieve bronchial problems.

In the case of coughs, the classic herbs are horehound, elecampane, and coltsfoot. These herbs reduce mucous secretions and soothe the bronchial passages. They can be added to the cold treatments just discussed if a cough arrives on top of the cold. If these herbs are combined with licorice and ginger, their effectiveness is increased because their power is spread better throughout the lungs, chest, and body.

FEVERS

In the case of influenza, or viral fevers in general, it is

important to know how to use ginger. You should take ginger at the stage of the fever when you are shivering or have cold hands and feet, and are experiencing a sensation of chill. Ginger can help the uncomfortable, restless, low-grade fever that does not "break" but rather seems to just drag on. Fresh ginger, grated into a drink with honey and lemon, can help to bring out the fever—bring the heat out from the center of the body to the periphery, to warm the hands and feet, to create sweating, and to hasten the "crisis," as it used to be called. The "crisis" is the point at which sweating is profuse, the temperature suddenly drops, and you feel much better. Ginger should not be used if the fever is high, you feel hot, or you are red and sweating.

Ginger used properly hastens natural healing. As you can see, it is used in the opposite manner of medications such as acetaminophen, which suppress fever and allow an illness to linger without a full cure.

Fever is not something to fear. It is the body's natural defense reaction, for the high temperature not only mobilizes the immune system but also inhibits the multiplication of viruses. The head is the part of the body most sensitive to fever. If necessary, apply cool wet towels to the head to control the fever or sponge the body with tepid water.

A thorough study of ginger's actions on fever has been carried out by Dr. N. Mascolo of the University of Naples in Italy working with colleagues at the University of Rajasthan in India. These researchers found that ginger is able to lower body temperature in animals that have fevers but does not affect their temperature when it is normal. In fact, it was nearly as effective as aspirin. The researchers suggested that ginger works somewhat like aspirin in that it reduces the production of prostaglandins (see Chapter 2). Of course, ginger is not the same as aspirin, and these studies are a great oversimplification, but this is a beginning.

RHEUMATIC PROBLEMS

The stiffness, slowness, and pain that result from rheumatic conditions are all regarded in Oriental medicine as being due to the entry of cold and dampness into the body, something well known to rheumatism sufferers, who are very sensitive to the weather. The whole process of the joints losing their lubrication, function, and warmth is seen as a cooling of the body, or, as Westerners say, atrophy. Ginger is one of the classic remedies for these conditions and is used both internally and externally. Since heat is needed near the surface of the body, fresh ginger is preferable, although dried ginger is also used.

In China, tea made of fresh ginger is drunk for all rheumatic complaints. Ginger is also mixed with other medicines or is injected by doctors at the site of the rheumatic joint or into nearby acupuncture points. Ginger poultices are another method. A clinical trial at the Guangdong Province Research Centre into Medicinal Plants tested the injection method with 113 patients suffering from rheumatic problems or chronic backache. A small amount was injected every other day into the region around the rheumatic joint. There were some burning sensations, numbness, and pain, but these soon subsided. The injections resulted in considerable improvement in the pain, swelling, and stiffness in more than 90 percent of the rheumatic patients. It was less effective for the patients with backaches. Of the 38 patients with rheumatic arthritis, 14 were cured, another 14 witnessed a considerable improvement, and 6 more showed some improvement. The remaining 4 were not helped.

Most people, of course, would not want fresh ginger injected into their joints, and in any case, this should be done only by a qualified practitioner. You can achieve significant improvement just by taking ginger orally. A report written by Dr. Srivastava (see page 21) and published in the journal *Medical Hypothesis* describes seven patients with rheumatoid arthritis who were greatly helped by taking fresh ginger by mouth. The average dose was about one ounce daily.

The treatment of rheumatic conditions is not simple, whether through herbs, homeopathy, or conventional medicine. Many remedies are potentially useful, depending on the patient, the nature of the rheumatic problem, and the stage of the disease. In Indian medicine, rheumatic problems are seen as the result of toxic accumulations, or Ama. Treatment is designed to clear these toxins from the body and includes mild laxatives and liver-strengthening remedies. The liver is targeted because it is the great housecleaner of the body. Ginger, galangal, and other spices are used to increase the patient's Agni, or fire, to burn up the toxic accumulations. Turmeric is also used because it has additional anti-inflammatory properties.

Other herbs are used to treat the bones and joints and to improve flexibility and lubrication. One of the most important in Ayurvedic medicine is guggul, known to us as *Commiphora mukul*, a resinous plant and a relative of myrrh. The plant is boiled with other herbs to make a compound herbal resinous tablet, which is commonly used in Ayurveda for treatment of arthritic and rheumatic problems, as well as conditions such as atherosclerosis.

In Western herbalism, the same principles are followed when cleaning out the body—the digestion is regulated and the liver is recharged. Herbs such as dandelion and burdock are used. As in Ayurveda, celery seed, parsley seed, juniper, nettle, and similar items are used to remove deposits from the body and to increase circulation and urination. Devil's claw, yucca, nettle, black cohosh, and meadowsweet are a few of the herbs used to treat the condition itself. They are often combined with cayenne or ginger.

MENSTRUAL PROBLEMS

Almost any health problem that involves stagnant energy, and especially stagnant fluids in the body, can be helped by ginger. Ginger is especially appropriate when the congestion or clogging does not involve an acute, serious health problem but just a general lowering of health.

Menstrual problems are such an instance. Menstruation is a good indicator of general health because any disruption in the normal, balanced flow of energy or fluids will show up there. Menstruation can be regular and without pain, discomfort, cramps, tension, headache, or emotional outbursts. Alternatively, as is very often the case, it can be scanty, irregular, excessive, late, or accompanied by the range of symptoms loosely lumped together as premenstrual syndrome (PMS). PMS can include tension, emotional upset, swollen breasts, tiredness, irritability, and all the symptoms described above.

The causes of menstrual problems may well be the same as those that disrupt harmony in other bodily systems—overwork, stress and anxiety, and too much fat, sugar, and starch in the diet, with too few minerals and vitamins. Degraded purified oils and animal foods are particularly suspect.

Ginger, turmeric, basil, and vervain are used as mild remedies for what the Chinese call "stuck," or "stagnant," blood. They all are effective in getting the blood moving to encourage regular, easy menstruation. In addition, they are mild. Chinese angelica, or Tang kuei, is the main Oriental herb in this category, and it is widely used by Oriental women and increasingly by Western women. Stronger Western herbs also exist, such as rue, pennyroyal, and motherwort, but they should not be used indiscriminately (preferably, they should be taken with the guidance of a qualified professional).

Again, take your constitution into account. Menstrual problems that are "watery" in nature—that is, Kapha in type—include swollen breasts, edema, heaviness, tiredness, weeping, and mucous discharge. They can be successfully treated with pungent spices such as ginger. Vata-type menstrual problems include irregularity and scantiness, as well as mood swings, instability, anxiety, pain, and headache. Gentle spicy remedies—such as aromatic herbs, chamomile, mint, Tang kuei, dill, turmeric, licorice, and a little ginger—will work here. Fire (Pitta) type problems include sweating, heat and hot flushes, rashes, abundant flow, and anger, and more cooling emmenagogues (blood-moving agents) are required, such as skullcap, yarrow, motherwort, calendula, and dandelion.

Clearly, ginger's warming effect on the body, its "internal sauna," is not just a pleasant experience for the tissues. The sauna effect can help mobilize our immunity and our body defenses, which in turn can mean faster recovery from a variety of infections, from the common cold to chronic bronchial problems. It can open vessels and bring healing fluids to places that have closed down and atrophied, thus helping rheumatic and arthritic problems in particular. It can keep the current of liquids moving properly in the body, helping problems such as menstrual irregularities. These are some of the more subtle and yet powerful effects of ginger, which are well known in traditional medicine and will now, hopefully, come to be enjoyed by many more of us.

CHAPTER 5

Growing and Trading
of Ginger

You may never have seen fresh ginger. Although it is becoming more common in our supermarkets, ginger, to many people, is little more than some brownish yellow powder, smelling of dust and pungency, in a plastic bottle that has been sitting in the kitchen spice rack since time immemorial.

Fresh ginger is an extraordinary sight. It is fleshy and bulbous and looks rather like several small potatoes clumped together and then flattened. The main segment is about three inches long, one-and-a-half inches wide, and a half-inch thick. It bears fat branches on the upper side that are about eight inches long, giving it the appearance of a hand with blunt, stubby fingers. Indeed, the technical terms for a piece of fresh ginger are "hand" for the whole piece and "fingers" for the branches. Fresh ginger has a smooth, corky skin that is buff or creamy brown and covers juicy white flesh.

THE GINGER PLANT

Botanically speaking, ginger is not a root. It is an underground stem, known as a rhizome, that bears buds on the top of each of its stubby fingers and grows a mass of thin, tangled roots below. The roots are scraped off before the ginger arrives in the supermarket, so we do not see them and often make the mistake of thinking that the rhizome itself is the root.

Under suitable conditions of dampness and temperature, the buds sprout. First comes a rolled-up green tube, which opens out as a stem—or, more accurately, as a pseudo-stem, since the ginger hand itself is the underground stem. The aboveground pseudo-stem can be three to four feet tall and bears blade-shaped leaves that branch out, ladderlike, on either side.

Ginger does not usually bloom, but when it does, it produces an exceptionally beautiful cluster of white or yellow flowers flecked with purple, each held in a small green cup. The cluster sits on a long, spiky stem, somewhat like a gladiolus.

Fresh ginger, when cut, produces a warm, spicy, refreshing aroma. Its taste is pungent, aromatic, lemony, and slightly bitter. Dried ginger is less fresh and lemony, rather more warm, woody, and pungent. Dried ginger is a shriveled version of a hand of fresh ginger. Pieces of it are hard, small, and flattened, having lost 80 percent of their weight and size in the drying process.

THE GINGER FAMILY

The botanical name for ginger is *Zingiber officinale* Roscoe. Ginger belongs to the family *Zingiberaceae*, as do many hundreds of other plants, some of them quite important to people. First are the plants that are botanically very close to ginger—that is, different types of ginger that belong not only to the family *Zingiberaceae* but also to the *Zingiber* group within it. One is *Zingiber cassumunar*, known in India as forest ginger. It is widely used in Indian medicine for diarrhea and colic and as a substitute for real ginger. In Thailand, it is used very widely as a flavoring spice, with an odor and taste similar to that of ginger but more camphoraceous and musty. The plant looks very much like true ginger, with a similar rhizome, which has a rich yellow interior. In Thailand, the plant is known as phlai, which probably has produced a few chuckles about Thai phlai.

Another type of ginger, *Zingiber zerumbet*, is widely cultivated throughout Asia, mostly as a medicine for coughs, asthma, stomachaches, and colic. In addition, unlike true ginger, it seems to be very popular for skin diseases. It tastes and smells like a bitter version of ginger, but its underground parts—its rhizome and roots—are gigantic. *Zingiber mioga* is the Japanese ginger, grown and used on that island nation instead of real ginger. However, it is so similar to the real thing that no one in the spice trade bothers to differentiate it botanically from the ginger grown in India and elsewhere. It is therefore usually lumped together with the official ginger, even though its flavor is much fruitier, more like bergamot. *Zingiber elatum* and *Zingiber chrysanthum* are other species of very aromatic Asian gingers.

A little farther removed—not a brother, but a cousin of ginger—is turmeric, *Curcuma longa*. As a plant, turmeric looks very similar to ginger. Indeed, if you saw a dried rhizome, you might think it was ginger. However, turmeric is far less aromatic than ginger, and it has a deep yellow color when dried and is bright orange when fresh. Turmeric is an exceedingly important Indian spice and medicine. It really deserves a book on its own. One of its key uses in India is as an antibacterial skin treatment. Made into a paste, it is placed on all kinds of skin infections and eczema. It draws out boils and ulcers, and it is generally the first-aid remedy of choice for minor cuts and wounds in traditional Indian households. Every little roadside stall in India offers turmeric soap, some of which is scented with sandalwood, which is the least expensive and most popular available. It is infinitely preferable to synthetic white supermarket soap, and it is about a tenth of the price. Turmeric's antiseptic properties are also useful in food. It prevents food from spoiling and also helps treat stomach infections due to bad food or water.

The main active ingredient in turmeric is a yellow compound called curcumin. This compound, along with turmeric itself, has been found to be strongly anti-inflammatory. It makes turmeric one of the best anti-inflammatory herbs known, a gentle herbal rival to cortisone. Turmeric is used internally for injuries, gallstones, dysmenorrhea, and inflammations of the urogenital system. It also helps improve liver function. In many ways, turmeric is a non-pungent version of ginger, for it seems to act similarly on the prostaglandins but does not have ginger's warming properties.

Another well-known relative of ginger is cardamom, or *Elettaria cardamomum* Maton. Cardamom's leaves are long ovals with prominent ribs, very similar to those of turmeric. However, in the case of cardamom, the seeds, not the rhizome, form the spice. Cardamom has a very special and exquisite aroma. It used to be called the "queen of spices." Cardamom is also used as a medicine, and it is extremely popular in the West as an essential oil. It is gently warming, removing gas, relieving indigestion, and reducing mucus in the stomach and lungs.

Several cheaper substitutes for classic cardamom also exist, although they are not usually found in the West. One is the wonderfully named grains of paradise, or *Amomum melegueta*. Others are *Amomum subulatum* and *Amomum aromaticum*, which are usually known simply as large cardamom or, sometimes, simply as amomum. Both these plants are spicy and have aromas like that of cardamom, just a little rougher.

The ginger family also includes a number of plants that are more medicinal than culinary, although they are used for both purposes. One is galangal, which is actually two plants—greater galangal (*Alpinia galanga*) and lesser galangal (*Alpinia officinarum*). Galangal may be more familiar to some people as China root. It is somewhat like ginger root when dried, but reddish and rounded. It has a sweet, aromatic smell. It has been well known and used in Europe for over 1,000 years, presumably brought by the Arabs, who introduced many herbs to Europe. It is still used in India, the Baltic states, and the Middle East to make aromatic herb teas and beers. In the Galilee hills, where I now live, the Druze and Arabs traditionally give a tea heavily spiced with galangal to women after childbirth. I have been presented with galangal tea several times when attending the celebration for the birth of a child. Medicinally, galangal has uses very similar to those of ginger.

Zedoary, or *Curcuma zedoaria*, is similar to turmeric. It is gray in color, with a bitter but aromatic taste, and it is used as a stomach remedy. Since the Middle Ages, it has been a constituent of a number of bitters that have stimulated jaded appetites and treated dyspeptic European tummies.

HOW TO GROW GINGER

Those of you braving the winter winds in the northern United States, Canada, Britain, and northern Europe will have to make do with your local supermarket, vegetable store, or Oriental food market for a supply of fresh ginger to keep you warm. This is because ginger is a hot-weather crop, growing best in countries such as India, Australia, Jamaica, China, and Nigeria. It cannot tolerate frost. However, my colleague, the late John Blackwood, grew ginger very successfully indoors in southern England, so if you can escape the cold with a greenhouse or a sunny or heated conservatory, you may be able to grow ginger even in a northern clime.

The ginger plant also does not like too much heat and will not grow in tropical or desert conditions. It does best when the climate is hot and moist and it can find at least a little shade from the direct glare of the noonday sun. It also likes to be in moist soil. Mulching helps to keep the top layers of the soil from drying out and damaging the sensitive roots near the surface. This is why ginger, as a rain-fed crop, is planted at the beginning of the monsoon season in India. In other places, it is well irrigated.

Ginger can be planted in late summer. Take a ginger hand and split it into half-ounce pieces; make sure each piece has a good, fat bud on it. Plant the ginger pieces in raised beds or mounds, about four to six inches into the soil and ten inches apart. The earth should be loose and rich, with plenty of organic material and compost. Ginger feeds heavily, exhausting soil of its nitrogen, potash, and minerals. Put a good mulch over the ground after planting the ginger pieces and add more as necessary. Soon after planting, you will see long, spiky leaves appearing and unrolling more or less in front of your eyes.

After six months, ginger can be harvested. Some very interesting research has been carried out on the correct time to harvest ginger. Ginger was found to mature in the soil the way carrots and radishes do, becoming stronger in flavor and more fibrous as time goes on. If harvested early, it yields a succulent, tender ginger that is aromatic, lemony, and mildly flavored. This is the tender "green" ginger that is harvested commercially for sale as fresh ginger or for making ginger sugar syrups. Waiting a couple of months allows the flavor to become stronger as more of the pungent components build up in the flesh of the ginger. The ginger is then a little drier and more fibrous. Commercially, it is harvested at this time for drying and selling as the full-flavored and pungent dried whole ginger. The latest harvest, at around nine months, yields the strongest ginger of all, richest in pungent components and quite dry. This ginger is used commercially for drying and then grinding as powdered ginger.

Ginger has some diseases that it must fend off, although these diseases are more of a problem in intensive agriculture than with pots in a conservatory. Like many root crops, ginger is susceptible to fungi that cause root rot, in which the ginger rhizome becomes soft and rotten. Little can be done in such cases other than to dig up the affected plants and burn them. It is best to protect against root rot by using the cleanest possible ginger for seed and by washing it with fungicide before planting. In addition, yellowing of the leaf may occur, as it does with potatoes and tomatoes, but again, this is a fungal problem, which can be treated with a safe fungicide.

If we took a journey to southwest India, to the rich, gently sloping farmland of Kerala state, and visited a ginger farm, what would we see? We would see several small fields of an acre or so. They would be growing tapioca and chilies, lines of little green bushes flecked with scarlet pods, or sesame, tall and stout, with an exquisite purple flower. One of the fields would have many raised beds, each about three feet wide and surrounded by a narrow drainage channel. The soil would be very richly manured, dark, and crumbly. In March or April, we would see the farmer, dark-skinned and wearing a colored *lungi* (short wraparound cloth), and his wife and family, dressed in bright and spotlessly clean *saris* (dresslike wraparound cloths), digging holes and planting pieces of ginger about a hand's width apart. Soon after the planting was finished, the farmer would lay down a dressing of fertilizer. Then, the children would spread a mulch of green leaves all over the beds to keep in the moisture and prevent the soil from being washed away by heavy rain. Occasionally after that, on dry days, the entire family would come out to weed the beds by hand or to pile up the earth around the bases of the tall, spiky ginger plants with a hoe. Come December, we would see the field take on a yellow hue, as the ginger tops began to dry up. The farmer would be out again with his family, carefully lifting out the ginger in clumps using a spade and putting it in baskets. The women would then carry the ginger to a shed and wash it.

If you can provide the right conditions, ginger is not difficult to grow, and it is well worth the effort, especially if fresh ginger is hard to find in your area. I enjoy growing ginger, watching the spiky leaves unfurl day by day and thinking of those heady flavors maturing under the earth. Here in Israel, in our Mediterranean climate, it does well—if we can stop the cats from digging it up first!

THE GINGER TRADE

On a recent visit to India, I traveled up the famed Malabar Coast, passing through towns whose names were made famous by the spice trade—Quilon, Allepey, Calicut, Cochin. In this last town, wandering through the small streets, I was repeatedly jostled as people hurried and scurried by, carrying spices, in a scene that must have been replayed on a daily basis for thousands of years. *Coolies*, or unskilled laborers, dark-skinned and intense, trotted back and forth with sacks on their backs. Simple bamboo carts passed, pulled by bright-eyed, shouting boys. Surrounding warehouses were piled to the ceiling with jute sacks bulging with aromatic contents. And quiet but sharp middlemen sat behind sample jars and watched over everything.

Who would believe that the Malabar Coast would currently be exporting some 15,000 tons of ginger per year? Much of this ginger goes to Europe, the traditional market. An average European consumes one ounce of dried ginger per year. An average American consumes one-half ounce per year. But only a tiny proportion of all the ginger that comes into the United States and Europe ends up on kitchen spice shelves. Most of the 5,000 tons of dried ginger imported annually into America goes to the bakery industry for the production of ginger biscuits and cakes, and substantial amounts go to other food industries to be processed into meat products, soups, pickles, and chutneys. In addition, the market for ginger in soft drinks is growing, and a little bit of ginger is still going to the pharmaceutical industry, especially for use in throat and cough preparations.

Now, let us trace ginger back to its sources and see what happens to it from there. As already mentioned, ginger is grown in several areas of the world, with total production around 100,000 tons. The ginger from each different area has its own individual flavor and texture, as well as its own local traditional method of preparation for market. Table 5.1 shows the main variations according to source.

FORMS OF GINGER

As just explained, when ginger is to be sold fresh, it is harvested early. Apart from trimming off the roots and cleaning the rhizome, the farmers do little to it before sale. Most of this green ginger is used in cooking in the countries

Table 5.1. Differing Characteristics of Ginger According to Origin

Source	Appearance	Taste
INDIA		
Cochin (unbleached)	Light brown, roughly peeled	Lemony, rooty, fairly pungent
Calicut (unbleached)	Reddish brown, roughly peeled	Fairly lemony, rooty, fairly pungent
Cochin/Calicut (bleached)	White, lime coated	Sweet, rooty, fairly pungent
AFRICA		
Nigeria	Dark, wrinkled, partly scraped	Camphoraceous, harsh, aromatic, rooty, strongly pungent
Sierra Leone	Very dark gray-brown, wrinkled	Earthy, camphoraceous, very pungent
JAMAICA	Light buff, smooth, hard, clean peel	Delicate, aromatic, spicy, mildly pungent
CHINA	Pale brown, unpeeled	Lemony, aromatic, mildly pungent
AUSTRALIA	Light brown, unwrinkled	Strongly lemony, fairly pungent

in which it is grown. Indeed, India itself uses at least 50,000 tons per year in this form. Some of this ginger is kept for preservation in sugar and syrup. In the West, very little green ginger is sold, with most of it going to the immigrant communities, where it can be found in local vegetable shops, ethnic markets, and, of course, Chinese and Indian restaurants. Some of this form of ginger is used in pickles and chutneys.

The most ginger by far is shipped from the growers already dried. Dried ginger is what most people know, for this is the pungent buff-colored powder in our spice jars. After the fresh ginger is harvested, it is washed and its roots are scraped off. It is then laid out on clean floors and dried in the sun for a week to ten days. During this time, it is turned occasionally and piled up every night. If the fresh ginger was too fleshy and moist, the drying will take longer and the ginger will end up looking shriveled. This is one of the reasons ginger for drying is harvested later, when it has lost more of its water.

Dried ginger is much stronger in taste and more pungent than fresh ginger. This extra strength is the result not only of the later harvest, which gives the plant more time to accumulate flavors, but also of the drying process, which seems to increase the pungent substances while reducing those that are lemony and aromatic. There is some evidence that even when dry, the rhizome grows somewhat more pungent during short-term storage, although if ground and stored for an extended period, it loses pungency. Clearly, this dried, wrinkled, dead-looking plant is alive and kicking somewhere inside.

In some villages, ginger is first soaked overnight and rubbed clean. Then, before drying, the corky outer skin is peeled off by hand with a sharp knife to produce a clean and smooth dried ginger of superior quality. The peeling has to be done carefully, however, as the tissues that contain the aromatic essential oil lie just under the skin and rough peeling can drastically reduce the aroma and taste. Hand-peeling is still done in Jamaica and in Kerala, India, but it is a disappearing skill and unnecessary if the dried ginger is to be ground into powder.

Today, the food and beverage industries often need a more concentrated ginger flavor. Adding ground ginger to a soft drink results in a muddy, turbid product. Therefore, ginger is extracted and concentrated. This also cleans the ginger of bugs and dirt. One way to extract dried ginger uses a solvent such as alcohol or acetone (nail polish remover). The fibrous residue is thrown away, and the solvent is carefully vaporized off under a vacuum, leaving a thick paste. This thick paste, called oleoresin, contains most of the flavor of the original ginger packed into one-fifteenth of the weight. It is strong stuff—only small amounts need to be added to food products. Another way of concentrating ginger's flavor is to remove the essential oils. This is done by forcing steam through a mash of ginger, after which the oil is collected by distillation. The oil is highly concentrated—approximately one part oil is obtained from forty parts fresh ginger—but it is very aromatic, sweet rather than pungent, and full of flavor. It is popular for use in soft drinks, for example.

Another traditional way of preparing ginger is to preserve it in sugar. This produces that brown-sugary, aromatic, and spicy chocolate-covered sweetmeat, or the crystallized brown, tasty sliver on top of a cake. Sweet ginger pieces in sugar are known as crystallized ginger, or stem ginger. The brown syrup in which the pieces are bathed is known as ginger syrup. These ginger products have lost most of their medicinal ingredients and are therefore not effective as remedies. They are made in the Far East, where for centuries they have been the most popular form of sweet, and they are also produced in Australia.

The process of making ginger syrup starts with fresh ginger, which is diced and then cooked in acid to soften its fibers to allow the sugar to enter its tissues. The cooking turns the ginger brown, removes its aromatic oils completely, and reduces its pungency. The cooked ginger is then soaked in a hot sugar solution for several days, with the sugar syrup continually replaced and more ginger constantly added to make the mixture gradually more concentrated. This eventually produces a syrup containing diced ginger pieces. This syrup is exported and used in all kinds of pickles, jams, and marmalades, as well as packaged in decorative jars for the Christmas market.

How are candied crystallized ginger pieces made? If you have a sweet tooth and a strong imagination, you are invited to dream up all kinds of sticky processes. In fact, however, the procedure starts with the same ginger syrup. The syrup is drained off, leaving the ginger pieces, which are lightly washed and dried. The ginger pieces are then quickly dipped in a very thick sugar solution and immediately rolled in dry sugar several times. The result is mild-tasting, crystallized brown chunks that bear little resemblance to the original knobby, pungent ginger hands.

I invite you to use more than your imagination, however. I invite you to become a "hands-on" ginger expert. To start, check to see what kinds of ginger are available in your local stores. Try to identify where they come from and the differences between them. Try several preserved and dried forms of ginger. Try, even, to grow ginger indoors or, if your climate permits, outside. There are some pleasant surprises in store for you on your way to becoming a ginger connoisseur!

CHAPTER 6

Chemistry of Ginger

I t is always exciting to look inside a living plant, with its aromas and flavors, its strange effects on our bodies, and its odd peculiarities that are yet to be discovered. This is the role of natural-product chemists. These chemists attempt to learn about some special quality of a plant by analyzing its chemical constituents. Their tools are those of the chemistry laboratory, which today includes some very sophisticated computer-controlled processes with exotic-sounding names—for example, high pressure liquid chromatography, thin layer chromatography, gas chromatography, mass spectroscopy, and nuclear magnetic resonance.

To conduct an analysis, the chemist will distill the essential oil in the plant or will extract all the alcohol-soluble constituents. These liquids can contain up to hundreds of chemicals, which are separated into groups according to their molecular size or chemical nature by special "fractionation" equipment. The chemicals are then put through analytical equipment that creates a typical trace or pattern, which can be compared to that of known chemical compounds. In this way, single compounds can be identified. Often, unusual compounds are found that might be the cause of the unique property of the plant. If they are, they might lead to the discovery of a new medication, or a new flavor or odor.

In this chapter, we will look at the chemical makeup of ginger and see what components make it such a powerful remedy.

COMPONENTS OF GINGER

Fresh ginger, the same as any underground root or rhizome such as a potato or a carrot, consists mostly of water. About 80 percent of ginger's weight is water. Around 2.3 percent of ginger is protein, and about 1 percent is fat. Again as in a potato, the main solid component in ginger is carbohydrate, or starch, at around 12 percent. This percentage is greater the more mature the ginger is, with the greatest amount of carbohydrate contained in a piece of ginger that has spent the maximum amount of time in the ground. About 2.5 percent of ginger is fibrous material, which is also present in greater amounts in more mature ginger; and 1.2 percent is minerals, mainly calcium, phosphorus, and iron. The vitamin content, too, is nothing exceptional. A good supply of the B vitamins—particularly thiamine, riboflavin, and niacin—is combined with a healthy dose of vitamin C. However, since only small amounts of ginger are consumed, the nutritional content is unimportant relative to the nutrients contained in the rest of the diet. As mentioned in Chapter 1, ginger and other spices are not generally viewed as nutrients. Rather, they are seen as valuable because of their unusual non-nutritive components.

Dried ginger has only about 10 percent moisture, instead of 80 percent like fresh ginger. Therefore, dried ginger contains four to five times more solid constituents than fresh ginger does.

Now let us look at the special compounds that are found in ginger. These special compounds are divided into two groups and are found in two places within the rhizome. One group is the essential oil of ginger. This is an aromatic oily liquid that is found in tiny vessels just under the corky skin. It is called essential oil because historically it was thought to be the sap, or essence, of the plant, like the blood of an animal. This is the oil that is collected by distillation, the same way that oils of flowers are collected by perfumers and the oil in mint or thyme is released in the process of tea making. The second group is the oleoresin, mentioned in Chapter 5, which is located in specialized cells dotted around the fleshy interior of the rhizome in between the starch cells. This oleoresin is indeed resinous, and it can be extracted and concentrated only by using alcohol or a special solvent such as ether.

Before continuing this discussion, I must stress how all plants, even those of the same species, vary in the amounts of their components. Plants are not stamped from a mold. Ginger varies greatly according to where it is grown, what variety it is, how long it was in the soil, what agricultural methods were used, if it was scraped, how it was dried and processed, and so on. The main constituents, such as starch, can vary by 50 percent between varieties. The special constituents—the oil and the oleoresin—can vary by 100 percent. For example, the scraped ginger from Cochin that is coated with lime to improve its appearance is only 1.49 percent essential oil. Much of the original amount is lost in the scraping. African ginger, however, has twice this amount of oil, as the skin is left on and it is a strong-tasting variety to begin with.

Oil of Ginger

Essential oil of ginger is rich in a multitude of compounds, each of which contributes to ginger's characteristic flavor and aroma. No one is quite sure why plants make these aromatic substances, many of which are composed of very complicated chemicals requiring a lengthy production line in the plant cells. These aromatic substances could be used by the plant as protection against some insects, or to attract others, particularly bees and wasps, to pollinate their flowers. Or they may be present to deter goats and cattle, which seem to use these plants as medicine but not as food.

Some of the main compounds in oil of ginger are zingiberene, curcumene, bisabolene, sesquiphellandrene, pinene, myrecene, borneol, and farnesene. There are many others, too, perhaps thirty in all. A particular group of compounds called citrals—including geraniol, limonene, and neral—is interesting because its members give a citric, lemony aroma to the oil. However, these compounds are not present in the oil of dried ginger, something that we can confirm by ourselves—the ground ginger in our spice racks does not have a lemony smell. Since these compounds are present in fresh ginger, however, it seems that the process of drying ginger in the hot sun produces all kinds of chemical changes, the loss of the citrals being the most noticeable to us. The dried ginger from Australia and, to some extent, from Cochin are exceptions in that they have some lemony aroma preserved because of the special harvesting and drying methods used.

In fact, the aroma of the oil in ginger varies from place to place and even from harvest to harvest. Cochin oil is described as being sweet, warm, rooty spicy, and containing a distinct lemony note, while Nigerian oil is described as harsh, warm, rooty spicy, and distinctly camphoraceous, and Chinese oil is called mild, aromatic, rooty, and lemony. These differences in the aromas are reflected in the very large variations in the chemical mixes of the oils.

Oil also changes with time. Foods can change taste during storage, with our sensitive palates recognizing if they have become old. When ginger oil or dried ginger is stored, various components can change and react with others, and the taste will alter accordingly.

It is interesting that plants and flowers that contain essential oils do not have an infinite variety of chemicals to call upon. The number of chemicals found in the plant world is limited, and the same ones crop up again and again in completely different types of plants. The aromas and flavors that we experience from basil, geranium, orange, and ginger are the result of different selections and amounts of many of the same substances. For example, ginger oil contains pinene, geraniol, and limonene, which were discovered originally in the pine tree, geranium, and citrus, respectively.

Oleoresin

Distillation of an aromatic plant to produce an essential oil is a traditional process, known for millennia. During the last century, chemically pure solvents, such as alcohol, became available. In 1879, a scientist by the name of Thresh extracted oil from ginger with acetone, resulting in a brown liquid. When the acetone had dissolved away, he was left with a pungent, thick, brown, oily paste—the oleoresin. From this paste, he managed to obtain the first pure chemical from ginger, a pungent substance that he named gingerol. Forty years later, in Japan, Dr. H. Nomura made the next two major contributions to ginger chemistry, first finding the compound zingerone in the oleoresin and later finding another pungent compound, which he called shogaol, after *shoga*, the Japanese word for ginger.

Several flavor chemists have used more sophisticated methods in recent years to delve deeper into these substances. Among their discoveries is that gingerol is, in fact, a number of gingerols; it is a group of very similar substances described as (6)-gingerol, (8)-gingerol, and (10)-gingerol. The numbers refer to the lengths of the chains of carbon atoms on the sides of the molecules. These three gingerols compose about one-third of ginger's oleoresin. The other substances, shogaol and zingerone, are also found in groups of three, similarly described as (6)-, (8)-, and (10)-shogaol and (6)-, (8)-, and (10)-zingerone. Gingerol is the most pungent of the ginger constituents, followed by zingerone and then shogaol. It is interesting to note that, when stored, gingerol gradually changes to shogaol, which is not very different from gingerol. This is why ground ginger's pungency gradually drops as the spice sits aging at the back of the kitchen cupboard.

The oleoresin of ginger has other, lesser components, such as (6)-, (8)-, and (10)-paradol; (4)-, (6)-, (8)-, and (10)-gingediol; (6)-methylgingediol; (4)- and (6)-gingediacetate; and (4)- and (6)-hexahydrocurcumin. These contribute to but do not determine ginger's flavor or medicinal effects.

DIETARY AIDS IN GINGER

While ginger does not contribute a great deal to our nutrition, it does help us get the most out of our food. The main reason for this is that ginger's medicinal components act as longshoremen or stevedores, carrying the food across the stomach wall and unloading it into the circulation. However, one or two interesting additional components in ginger also help the diet. One is protease, which is present in a considerable amount. Protease is a catalytic substance similar to that used by the stomach to digest meat. As mentioned in Chapter 1, ginger is a good candidate for a commercial natural meat tenderizer. It certainly aids in the digestion of meat, which may be one of the reasons that the Chinese and other Asian peoples use it in meat dishes. Ginger also has a substance similar to protease, a lipase, which helps in the digestion of fats.

The other unusual components in ginger are antioxidants. Antioxidants are compounds that prevent foods from spoiling or becoming rancid. Chemicals such as butylated hydroxytoluene (BHT) are usually added to food products for this purpose. Ginger has been found to be the best of all the spices at preventing oxidation in food and is even stronger than BHT. If it can prevent oxidation in food, it may be able to do the same in our bodies. Oxidation in the body creates free radicals, destructive rogue chemicals that contribute to many degenerative diseases, such as atherosclerosis, and that hasten aging. It is not known for certain if ginger can do this, but scientists theorize that this action is partly responsible for ginger's ability to prevent the rise of cholesterol levels in the bloodstream. Cholesterol is more easily removed if it has not been oxidized.

MEDICINAL AIDS IN GINGER

The most exciting part of all this chemical dissection of ginger is that it facilitates exploration into how the plant's individual substances affect the body. By trying each of the substances in turn on, say, the stomach, it is possible to decide which one actually calms the tummy. Eventually, we may be able to catch a glimpse of how the various constituents act together to achieve the beneficial effects of the whole plant. This is never possible to do completely, however, as the whole effect results from the concerted, harmonious action of a very large number of contributing chemicals. Even with the most intensively researched plants, such as garlic, that goal is still far away. But we can make a start.

You may be wondering why we should bother with all this chemical interference. Indeed, the identification of single chemicals in plants does have a bad name among holistically and naturally minded folk. The main activity of the pharmaceutical industry seems to be taking a safe plant remedy, rich in therapeutic substances, and "boiling it down" to a little toxic white pill containing one single chemical. However, there is another practical purpose to learning about the chemistry of a plant besides getting out the king chemical and selling it. If we can discover which ingredients in plants are the main active ones, we can determine which varieties of plants are the best, as well as monitor the strength and consistency of plant remedies.

In the case of ginger, laboratory research has shown time and again that the main medicinal components are not in the starches, minerals, or water-soluble components, nor in the essential oil, but in the oleoresin. More than that, research has pinned down gingerols and shogaols as the main active components, with the others as minor contributors.

Scientists at Kyoto Pharmaceutical University in Japan have studied which components in ginger stop vomiting and nausea. The vomiting reflex is controlled by the stomach's nervous system, which uses a messenger called serotonin to kick the stomach into the powerful contractions we call vomiting. The Kyoto researchers discovered that ginger's oleoresin was much more effective than its oil in blocking this messenger. Dr. Johji Yamahara and colleagues went even further. They split the oleoresin into its components, tested each one, and determined that the gingerols were mainly responsible for getting in the way of the serotonin messenger.

Ten years earlier, this research team had come to similar conclusions concerning other actions of ginger. These scientists had found that the gingerols were responsible for ginger's ability to stimulate the gallbladder and the liver. Since the bile gland and liver are part of one of the main cholesterol-clearing routes in the body, the gingerols may also be ginger's cholesterol-reducing agents.

As we discussed in Chapter 2, ginger inhibits the manufacture of prostaglandins, which may be the way it warms the body and acts on the circulatory system. Researchers have shown that ginger has several compounds that are responsible for this and that some of them are gingerols. However, an additional series of substances in the oleoresin was also found to be highly active in this way—indeed, much more so than the chemical indomethacin, which is one of the strongest anti-inflammatory, prostaglandin-reducing medications available. This additional series includes the gingerdiones and dehydrogingerdiones. Interestingly, these are the chemicals that the plant cells use to make the gingerols. Therefore, the whole chain of pungent ginger substances may eventually be found to act together on the body.

Of course, this is not the whole story. There are situations in which other components of ginger besides the pungent ones probably come to the fore—for example, ginger oil assists in the treatment of colds and flu, for which sweating is needed. Obviously, the pungent components do not do everything. However, now that we know that they are of central importance, we can confirm scientifically that dried ginger is better than fresh for stomach problems, inflammation, and high cholesterol.

Another conclusion reached by the researchers is that the more pungent varieties of ginger are the more medicinal. This means that we should use African ginger or unpeeled Indian ginger. Peeling produces a nicer-looking rhizome but reduces the potency.

It is a peculiar fact that the *British Pharmacopoeia* always recommended Jamaican ginger for medicinal syrups and ginger cough mixtures. This ginger looks better and was commonly regarded as being of a higher quality. Medicinal ginger was even called Jamaica Ginger in some medical books. However, we now know that Jamaican ginger, though it looks better and is more expensive, is in fact medicinally less effective than other varieties. Perhaps the British Pharmacopoeia Commission should have consulted traditional herbalists rather than spice experts.

With our knowledge of the main active compounds in ginger, another door has opened. We can now check that those ingredients are actually present in a ginger product or preparation. Suppose you want to buy a bottle of ginger capsules or tablets. You could look at the label and read that the tablets contain ginger, but you would not be able to tell how strong the ginger is. The ginger could be weak or even have no medicinal components at all! You would simply have to trust the manufacturer. But until very recently, manufacturers had no idea. Until researchers isolated the medicinally active compounds, even the manufacturers of ginger products did not know what to look for when buying ginger to pack into tablets.

All this is now changing. Some manufacturers now realize that they must make sure that there are plenty of gingerols and other pungent components in their ginger products. If they do not have the analytical equipment to check this themselves, they ask their suppliers to do the analysis and to guarantee a certain ratio. It is therefore possible today to purchase ginger tablets and capsules containing known and fixed—that is, standardized—amounts of the gingerols. As a discerning ginger consumer, you should always look at the label of a ginger medicinal product to make sure that the manufacturer guarantees a given amount of gingerols in the product.

To get an idea of the richness of the substances in ginger, see Table 6.1. This table was prepared by Dr. James A. Duke, one of the world's leading experts on medicinal plants and a member of the United States Department of Agriculture. Dr. Duke's table shows just how many substances are found in ginger and some of their effects on our health. It indicates how the end result of taking ginger is a unique and complex action, a kind of symphony composed of the intermingling sounds of many separate instruments.

The ginger rhizome, like all plants, contains a very large number of different substances, many of which affect our bodies. This is very confusing, and even irritating, to people who believe that a medicine is a single, defined chemical, pure and of absolutely known dosage. But to those who prefer natural remedies, ginger's very complexity is the key to its value to humans. Its biologically active substances work on a variety of body systems, giving the plant its wide range of health applications—from colds to digestive problems. Moreover, the substances work together, helping each other and increasing each other's effectiveness. Also, the number of substances present makes the plant safe, since the different chemicals balance and soften each other. At the same time, there are two substances—gingerol and shogaol—that are the keys to ginger's effectiveness. This knowledge is important, for it helps us dis-

Table 6.1. Some Biologically Active Compounds in Ginger

Substance	Effect
Asparagine	Promotes urination.
Borneol	Analgesic, anti-inflammatory, lowers fever, protects liver.
Chavicol	Kills fungi.
Cineole	Anesthetic, clears chest/throat infections and coughs, antiseptic, lowers blood pressure.
Citral	Antihistamine, antibiotic.
Cumene	Narcotic.
Cymene	Antiflu, kills viruses, kills fungi, kills insects.
Dehydrogingerdione	Inhibits prostaglandins, treats liver.
Geraniol	Anticandida, kills insects.
Gingerdione	Inhibits prostaglandins.
Gingerol	Analgesic, lowers fever, stimulates circulation, lowers blood pressure, treats and calms stomach.
Hexahydrocurcumin	Treats liver, stimulates bile.
Limonene	Can irritate skin, deters insects.
Linalool	Anticonvulsive, antiseptic.
Myrecene	Kills bacteria, kills insects, muscle relaxant.
Neral	Kills bacteria.
Pinene	Removes phlegm, kills insects.
Shogaol	Analgesic, lowers fever, sedative, constricts blood vessels, raises blood pressure.
Zingerone	Raises blood pressure.

Source: Herbalgram 17 (Summer 1988), page 20. Used by permission of Dr. James A. Duke.

tinguish ginger that is medicinally effective from ginger that is less effective. So, by leaving all the chemicals in the plant, plus detecting and analyzing the main effective ones, we have the best of all worlds—a plant medicine that is safe and scientifically controlled in potency.

CHAPTER 7

History and Folklore of Ginger

Once there was a baker who made a beautiful gingerbread boy. He mixed a dough containing plenty of ground ginger, rolled it out, shaped it into a boy, and positioned raisins for the eyes and for the buttons on the boy's little waistcoat. He put the boy into a roaring oven. When the boy was done, he took him out on his baker's peel.

The gingerbread boy was crusty, nutty-brown in color, and sweet, rich, and aromatic. But as the baker stood admiring him, the boy looked up from the peel and hopped off. He glanced back, smiling impudently. "I am the gingerbread boy and you can't catch me," he teased. And off he ran, with the baker in pursuit, apron flapping in the breeze.

As the gingerbread boy ran through the village, a cat saw him and called out, "Stop! Stop!" for the boy smelled delicious. But the boy just ran on, shouting, "Run, run, as fast as you can; you can't catch me, I'm the gingerbread man!"

One by one, all the animals in the village and all the inhabitants of the village tried to catch and eat the gingerbread boy, but they could not overtake him. Then the boy came to a river. As he was deciding how to cross it, a fox came up.

"I'll take you across," the fox said.

"No, you'll eat me," said the gingerbread boy.

But the fox persisted, and by lies and whining pleas, he managed to persuade the gingerbread boy to ride on his back. In midstream, however, the fox promptly turned and finished the gingerbread boy off.

GINGER IN FOLKLORE

The story of the gingerbread boy is a well-known folktale, handed down from parents to children for many generations now. While all who hear it or tell it attach their own significance to the story, ginger aficionados find the tale to be a perfect description of the mercurial character of their favorite spice.

Ginger is aromatic and delicious, attracting everyone who catches a whiff of it as it passes by. It also moves very fast. It warms up everyone who takes it (or, in this tale, chases it), for they catch the same spirit of movement and are carried along by it. The tale is an allegory for ginger circulating through the body, moving quickly, overcoming obstacles, and warming up the system. Indeed, the image of a sleepy village waking up and running in circles could not be a clearer metaphor for a stimulated circulatory system.

Gingerbread houses are another prominent feature of some of our best-loved folktales. In "Hansel and Gretel," for instance, a gingerbread house is used by the evil witch to entice children into her dwelling. Here, the spicy aroma of ginger is equated with the eagerness and curiosity of youngsters, combined with the feeling that ginger is a homey spice that "makes all things nice" and cannot therefore represent harm or danger.

In England, gingerbread has always been popular. Queen Elizabeth I enjoyed it, and it has become traditional regional fare, acquiring different names in different localities. For example, in the early 1900s, it was called *feridge* in Norfolk, *lollybranger* in Somerset, and *parliament, scranchum,* or *thickels* in Northamptonshire. Gingerbread was important at country fairs and festivals. Gingerbread men were called husbands, with obvious reference to their warming qualities. Sometimes they were shaped like letters or given (to quote W. T. Fernie in *Kitchen Physic,* 1901) "whimsical devices, sometimes coarsely significant." This last item points to an erotic use for ginger.

Ginger, like other medicinal plants, has accumulated legends and folktales that back up humankind's belief in its medicinal powers. In traditional thought, all plants that help human beings were placed in the world by deities. They did not, as modern scientists insist, appear by accident. For example, among the tribal people of its homelands, ginger is regarded as a vehicle of magical force and power. In East Papua, Papua New Guinea, it is used to heat up the body before casting a spell. It is also chewed and spat out to ward off sudden squalls at sea, and spat into a precious cargo in a canoe to preserve it from harm. The anthropologist Bronislaw Malinowski, visiting the Trobriand Islands of Papua New Guinea from 1915 to 1918, found that the inhabitants there used a species of wild ginger in rituals connected with the harvest and the storage of food. These people would also spit ginger onto the roads entering their villages to deter misfortune and hunger and to encourage prosperity.

In medieval times, some people were so amazed at the wonderful aromas and tastes produced by ginger, and at its other benefits, that they believed the plant was a direct export from Paradise. In 1305, Sire Jean de Joinville traveled to Alexandria in Egypt with Saint Louis. His writings tell of the common belief of that time that the spices in Egypt came directly from the earthly Garden of Eden. The four great rivers—the Ganges, Tigris, Euphrates, and Nile—flowed around the Garden, according to folklore, and carried the spices that fell into them. Where the Nile re-emerged on the surface of the Earth, fishermen could stretch their nets in the evening and, in the morning, would sometimes find them "full of cinnamon, ginger, rhubarb, cloves, wood of aloes, and other such good things."

GINGER'S VENERABLE HISTORY

In 1972, the perfectly preserved tomb of the wife of the Prince of Tai was discovered in China. The princess had died shortly after 168 B.C. In the tomb were bamboo cases and pottery jars containing a large number of foodstuffs, including ginger and such other spices as cinnamon bark, pepper, and galangal. This discovery has provided some of the earliest evidence of the importance of ginger to the Orientals. Because of it, we can assume that in ancient times, ginger was as vital a part of the Oriental culture as it is today. Certainly, all the old Chinese herbals mention ginger, the best-known being the *Shen Nung Pen Tshao Tching*, or *Manual of the Celestial Husbandman*, a classic text recording a 5,000-year-old verbal tradition.

Confucius reportedly always liked to keep a dish of ginger by him when he ate. The earliest Chinese recipes, called the Eight Delicacies, were supposedly preserved from ancient times by Confucius, written down in the *Li*

Chi, or *Book of Rites*. One of these recipes reads: "To make the grill, they beat the beef and removed the skinny parts. Then they laid it in a frame of reeds, sprinkled on it pieces of cinnamon and ginger, and added salt. It could be eaten thus when dried. Mutton was treated in the same way as beef, and also the flesh of elk, deer and muntjac."

Literary evidence from the early centuries of the Christian era points to ginger being used as a seasoning for dried meat and fish, as were pepper, salt, and salted beans. During the Tang Dynasty (A.D. 618–907), venison seasoned with ginger and vinegar was first recommended by pharmacists in the *Shen Meng* and *Ts'ang-Ch'i Ch'en* as a tonic, but it later came to be valued for its taste as well.

The Chinese enjoyed ginger sweetened with honey. When Marco Polo visited China in early medieval times, he found honeyed and candied ginger being sold in the streets, especially at the onset of winter. In addition, the Chinese flavored tea with ginger and tangerine peel. Wine, which was generally made from rice or millet, was spiced with ginger or, sometimes, with pepper, chrysanthemum, pomegranate flowers, or saffron.

The Chinese were great traders across the China Seas and the Indian Ocean. The North African world traveler Ibn Battuta, writing in A.D. 1349, reported seeing their huge junks, with sails made of woven bamboo matting, in the harbor at Calicut, on the southwest coast of India. The sailors took their families with them on their two-year voyages and lived in comfortable quarters on board. "The sailors live in their cabins with their children. They grow herbs for cooking, vegetables and ginger in wooden tubs ... In all the universe there are no richer people than the Chinese."

Customs have not changed. Ginger is still used extensively in China, in much the same ways it was used in historical times. In the north, it is frequently an ingredient in sauces for meat and fish, while in the south, it is used more like a vegetable than a spice. Some cooks include it in all meat dishes. Ginger also plays a part in rituals. In Hong Kong, ginger is offered in the various temples. It is sometimes hung in huge paper constructions in the temples as an offering to the deity in an attempt to promote fertility.

In the West, ginger has been known as long as there has been trade with the East, which is a very long time. Ships sailed from the Malabar Coast of India to Arabian ports several thousand years ago. From these ports, spice caravans made their way up to Egypt. Such a caravan, with a crew of Ishmaelites, picked up Joseph and brought him to Egypt some 3,500 years ago. The spice trade across the Middle East is mentioned in the Bible many other times, too.

GINGER IN THE CLASSICAL AGE

Spices have always represented a measure of sophistication. Whoever could afford to flavor his food with exotic spices, usually brought at considerable expense from far away, was sure of his place in the superior classes. Thus, spices were sought after by all cultures. Empires, including the British Empire, were built on this quest for spices. Indeed, the search for new tastes and flavors has been one of the major forces behind human expansion and development. The ancient Romans were avid consumers of spices, as they were of all kinds of strange foods and medicines. They imported from the Middle East and India, either through Arab middlemen or by undertaking their own trading expeditions. Not every Roman supported this quest for the exotic, however. Gaius Pliny, known as Pliny the Elder, was one who disapproved, while at the same time giving us some interesting information about spices in his *Natural History*, written around A.D. 77. He wrote about ginger:

> The root of the pepper-tree is not, as some people have thought, the same as the substance called gingiberi, or by others zingiberi, although it has a similar flavor. Gingiberi is grown on farms in Arabia and Troglodytica; it is a small plant with a white root. The plant is liable to decay very quickly, in spite of its extreme pungency. Its price is six denarii a pound. It is remarkable that the use of pepper has come so much into favor. In the case of some commodities their sweet taste is their attraction, and in others their appearance, but pepper has nothing to recommend it in either fruit or berry. To think that its own pleasing quality is pungency and that we go all the way to India to get this! Who was the first person who was willing to try this on his food, or in his greed for an appetite was not content merely to be hungry? Both pepper and ginger grow wild in their own countries and yet they are bought by weight like gold and silver.

In Pliny's time, the Romans apparently imported their ginger from Yemen, located on the southwest coast of the Asian peninsula. Yemen was a fertile, well-watered land prior to the bursting of the great dam at Marib in the sixth century A.D. Around A.D. 150, Ptolemy spoke of ginger as being imported from Ceylon: "The products of Ceylon are rice, honey, ginger, the beryl, nakinthos, metals of all sorts including gold and silver, and elephants and tigers." Ginger appears in six recipes in the most famous Roman cookbook, written by Apicius in the fourth to fifth century

A.D. It was one of the few herbal medicines that Roman doctors carried with them when they accompanied the legions on their marches. They found or grew other herbs locally.

The spice trade did not cease with the fall of the Roman Empire. Churchmen continued to bring or send medicinal substances, including ginger, to England and Europe. In seventh- and eighth-century France, Marseilles was a key port for the import of spices, which were exempt from taxes by the Merovingian kings. In the ninth century, the monks of Corbie planned to buy numerous spices in the market in Cambrai, in northeast France, including pepper, ginger, cinnamon, galangal, myrrh, thyme, cloves, sage, and mastic. Then came the rise of Islam, and the Mogul emperors began governing the spice lands of the East. Arab traders held a monopoly over the spice trade for centuries.

ARABIAN NIGHTS

Ginger was always a strong presence in the Arab world. It appears in the Koran: 76, 15–17. In his younger days, Mohammed was a spice trader, and among Arab merchants, the dealers in spices were aristocrats because they traded in the exotic.

Many Arab merchants settled permanently on the southwest coast of India, the Malabar Coast, home to the great ports of Quilon, Cochin, and Calicut. These ports, as already described in Chapter 5, were the scenes of an extensive trade in ginger. Benjamin of Tudela, who traveled from Spain between 1160 and 1173, gave the following description:

> Thence it is seven days journey to Khulan [Quilon] which is the beginning of the country of

the Sun worshippers. These are the sons of Cush, who read the stars and are all black in color. They are honest in commerce. When merchants come to them from distant lands and enter the harbor, three of the King's secretaries go down to them and record their names and then bring them before the King. Whereupon the King makes himself responsible even for their property, which they leave in the open unprotected. Pepper is found in that country. They plant the trees thereof in their fields and each man of the city knows his own plantation. The trees are small and the pepper is white as snow. And when they have collected it they place it in saucepans and pour boiling water over it, so that it may become strong. Then they take it out of the water and dry it in the sun, and it turns black. Cinnamon and ginger and many other kinds of spices are found in this land.

Ginger appears often in Arabic poetry, and in the stories of *The Arabian Nights*, it is featured as an aphrodisiac. Anything that heats the blood can be an aphrodisiac, especially in the luscious, erotic world depicted in those stories.

GINGER IN EUROPE

Ginger has always been closely associated with pepper. During the centuries that the spice trade flourished between Asia and Europe, pepper was commonly the most important commodity, with ginger running second.

The history of ginger in the Middle Ages is the history of the spice trade, with the different routes to and from the East rising and falling in importance but always maintaining a healthy activity. These included the sea routes via Arabia to Europe and the great overland caravan routes through Turkey and Persia or through Turkestan and Russia. Spices were used to preserve and flavor foodstuffs. They were also utilized as medicines. They had great status value in society, and the prices for spices imported to Europe could reach high levels. Taxes were sometimes paid in pepper, as well as in ginger. In the town of Aix, in medieval France, the archbishop taxed the Jewish community in pepper, ginger, and wax for their right to have schools and cemeteries. In Basel, in medieval Switzerland, the street where the Swiss traders sold spices was called Imbergasse, which translates as Ginger Alley.

The search for the secret sources of the spices, which until that time had been controlled by the Arabs, was the reason the Portuguese and Spanish kings sent out Magellan, Vasco da Gama, Columbus, and many lesser-known explorers, who were the first ones to chart the globe. Around the beginning of the sixteenth century, the Portuguese controlled the oceans and therefore the rich pickings of the spice trade. They also conquered the Malabar Coast of India, in particular Goa. Within fifty years, the Spanish imported ginger to the West Indies, where it grew with even greater flavor and abundance. Then the Dutch, followed by the British, took over and dominated the Indian and Malaysian trade. Spices came up to London via the Suez Canal, and London became a major spice center. Dockside warehouses were stacked with the same aromatic cargo in gunny sacks that crowded the streets of Cochin.

Ginger appears again and again in English literature of all periods. It was a common household item, although it may have been reserved for special occasions. Chaucer, in *The Romance of the Rose*, describes a wonderful garden:

There was eke wexyne many a spice
As clowe-gelope, and lycorice,
Gyngevre, and greyn de Paradys,
Canell, and setewale of prys,
And many a spice delitable
To eten whan men arose fro table.

"Clowe," of course, is cloves; "canell" is cinnamon; and "setewale," later known as "setwall," is the old word for zedoary.

Shakespeare mentioned ginger several times. In *The Winter's Tale*, a feast is prepared and plans are laid to borrow "a race of ginger" from neighbors. In *Love's Labour Lost*, Costard announces, "And I had but one penny in the world, thou shouldn't have it to buy gingerbread." In *The Merchant of Venice*, Salanio quips, "I would she were as lying a gossip in that as ever knapped ginger." Ginger is "knapped," or snapped, into pieces. Is this the origin of the well-known gingersnaps?

A wonderful English use of ginger was to spice up beer or porter. For centuries, tavern keepers would place a jar of ginger on the bar for customers to help themselves. Beer was especially spicy when it was also warmed with a hot poker.

GINGER IN THE WESTERN HERBAL TRADITION

Herbalists in the West also respected and used ginger, although not to the extent that it was used in China and India, where the plant was indigenous. It all started, as you might have expected, with the Greeks, who acquired their ginger from Arab spice merchants and soon discovered its medicinal power. Pythagoras is said to have recommended it as a digestive aid and carminative. Galen, the true father of modern medicine, was impressed with ginger's heating properties: "It creates heat powerfully, but not immediately at first contact like pepper." In other words, ginger generates a fire that is more gentle but also longer lasting.

In ancient Rome, ginger was one of the ingredients of the Mithridatius, a compounded remedy created by the physicians to King Mithridates VI around 80 B.C. as a protection against poisoning. It became one of the Four Official Capitals, or four main remedies, of the Roman period.

European herbalists all looked back to the classical period for instruction and inspiration, to which they added their own discoveries. The most famous Renaissance herbalist, Gerard, wrote: "Ginger, as Dioscorides reporteth, is right good with meat in sauces, or otherwise in conditures; for it is of an heating and digestive qualitie, and is profitable for the stomacke, and effectually opposeth it selfe against all darkness of the sight ..." Gerard actually tried to grow ginger in England, but he sadly reported that it was killed by frost. Presumably, he did not have the benefit of a conservatory with a sunny southern exposure.

The classical period was also the high point for Arabic medicine, and naturally, since the Arabs were the spice merchants of Europe, ginger figured prominently in their medicine chests. According to *The Medicine of the Prophet*, a guide written by Al Sayuti of Cairo in the latter part of the fifteenth century:

> Ginger is hot and dry in the third degree, and dry in the second. It contains [prevents] excess of damp. It is an aid to digestion, strengthens sexual intercourse and dissolves wind. If the purge Turbith [a common medieval laxative] is weak, or if there is oedema, then its reaction is strengthened by the addition of ginger. It renders fluid the

thickness of phlegm. A confection of ginger soothes the stomach. It is a help in old age.

In Chapter 4, we mentioned that King Henry VIII, in one of his many regal manias, insisted that the Lord Mayor of London use ginger against the plague. Henry was not the only royal personage with a ginger obsession. Queen Elizabeth I had a famous "pother," or powder, which was comprised mainly of white ginger, along with cinnamon, caraway, anise, and fennel powders. She took this remedy "at anietime after or before meate, to expel winde, comfort ye stomach, and help digestion."

We can recognize in these traditional uses the same themes we have discussed in previous chapters, themes that are mostly confirmed by modern research—ginger warms the body, improves and stimulates the circulation, and helps the stomach. Some beneficial consequences can also be seen—better circulation and body function in old age and improved sex life. These are obviously linked to body heat and circulation. We even describe a sexually active person as "hot blooded."

GINGER IN THE UNITED STATES

Ginger does not have a long history in the United States. Early Native Americans did know of it, and there are indications that the Creeks used it at one time to promote sweating in an effort to rid the body of infection. However, Native Americans tended to use another plant for the uses described in this book. That plant was wild ginger, given its name because of its gingerlike properties and taste. However, wild ginger, better known as Canadian snakeroot, bears no relation to real ginger.

The history of real ginger in the United States goes back

to the time the Spanish brought the spice from India and began to plant it in their colonies in the West Indies. The ginger grown in the West Indies, especially in Jamaica, was of good quality. Indeed, until recently, Americans imported all their ginger from Jamaica. It even came to be called Jamaica ginger by the early settlers and herbalists, who probably introduced it to the Native Americans. A fluid extract of Jamaica Ginger was listed in American pharmacopoeias as an aid to digestion and was widely sold in the young country, where it became known as jake.

However, a notorious episode involving Jamaica ginger occurred during Prohibition. In 1930 and 1931, thousands of people were poisoned by jake, or, rather, by the 70-percent alcohol it contained. Jake was one of the only alcohol-containing liquids that could be legally purchased during Prohibition. But the alcohol used to make it was often contaminated, and many of the people who drank a bad batch became permanently semiparalyzed. Jake is no longer sold in the United States, although several American blues songs have immortalized it.

HISTORY OF THE WORD "GINGER"

The word "ginger" has passed largely unaltered through the Indo-European languages—that is, the languages of the European group including Greek and Latin. In Greek, ginger is *ziggiberis*; in Latin, *zingiber*; in French, *gingembre*; in Spanish, *jenjibre*; in German, *Ingwer*; and in English, *ginger*. All of these derive from the Sanskrit, which is the mother of the Indo-European languages. The Sanskrit word for ginger is *sringa-vera*, meaning "antler-shaped," which in turn comes from a Dravidian root, a prehistoric form of Malayan, in which ginger is *inchi-ver*. In Arabic, ginger is *zanjabil*, and in Hebrew, *zangvill*. These languages have a Mesopotamian or Egyptian root. However, in the case of ginger, they borrowed the term, along with the spice itself, from the East.

In modern Hindi, ginger is known as *Ada*, or *Adrak*; it is *Adrakam* in related dialects. However, these names apply to fresh ginger only. Dried ginger is *Sunthi*.

Clearly, ginger has a rich and varied history, to match its wide use as a medicine and a food. It might help some people to better accept ginger as a valuable remedy if they realized that the history and folklore of such a plant were natural parts of our culture. There is no reason for a medicine to be a mysterious drug that ordinary people cannot understand or that has a name ordinary people cannot pronounce. A medicine does not have to stand above people or outside their literature and legend. Rather, stories and tales and history can provide a kind of background knowledge for ordinary people to use to become familiar with, and come to love, natural remedies. They make natural remedies such as ginger "user friendly."

CHAPTER 8

Ginger Products
and Preparations

We know by now that ginger is not one "thing" that we take for one particular health problem. It is a symphony of varied chemical ingredients that changes all the time, depending on its origin, its form, and its method of preparation. This means that every ginger rhizome is slightly different from every other one. And if we vary the method of preparation, the dosage, and the source, we can obtain a different chemical cocktail that has somewhat different biological effects. Ginger can therefore be useful for a number of health problems.

In this chapter, we will look at the various traditional ways of preparing and taking ginger, and we will discuss how these preparations can be used for different purposes. We will also examine how we can make sure we are getting our money's worth—that is, how we can ascertain that we have potent, good-quality ginger for use as a medicine.

BUYING GINGER PRODUCTS

Little doubt exists that, in general, the best way to take an herb is in its fresh and unprocessed state. When I need to use a particular herb, I go out into my garden and pick the leaves or root, which I then use right away. These are the times I thank my lucky stars for the investment in labor that I have made in my herb garden, since I know what I am getting. If you go to a store and buy an herb—as either dried leaves or tablets—you have to trust that they are of the correct species because you have no way of knowing for sure. You also have to trust that the leaves or tablets are still sufficiently fresh and have not lost any active components through age. You do not know if the herb was grown in the best way or if it is of the most medicinally active variety. It might also be contaminated or lower in dosage than the packaging states.

You might contend that a reputable supplier of herbal remedies would not monkey with the herbal stock. This is true. But the problem is that many suppliers of herbal products do not themselves have the technical ability to analyze and check that the herbs they purchase are really top quality. For example, a shipment of ground ginger arriving from the East may look exactly as it should. Yet someone in the Far East may have already extracted some of the active ingredients, leaving mostly residue. This does happen, and only laboratories have the equipment to detect it. For example, many feverfew tablets sold in North America have little in the way of active ingredients. This is because the wrong variety of feverfew herb is generally used. The right and wrong plants look exactly the same. Again, only a laboratory can tell.

With ginger, we are a little better off because the active ingredients can actually be tasted. These ingredients are the pungent components, so if ginger tastes pungent, it is probably good. We are not so fortunate with other herbs. You would have to be a real herbal expert to taste the difference between good and bad batches of ginseng, echinacea, and, indeed, most herbs.

It is also easier to make sure you are getting the correct plant if you can see the rhizome. This, obviously, is not possible with powder. Ground ginger does get adulterated with substances like flour and chalk. In an investigation by the Inland Revenue in Ottawa, Canada, 150 samples of ground ginger were tested in a laboratory. Of these, 21 were adulterated and 14 were doubtful. Even adulterated ginger, or ginger that has had its soluble ingredients removed, can taste pungent, for someone has come up with the mean trick of adding hot pepper powder to ginger residue to make it seem pungent. Another problem is that ginger and medicinal foods are occasionally full of bacteria, fungi, or even insects. If they are not, they may contain the chemical residues of the treatments that killed the bacteria, fungi, and insects, which are probably worse.

Where does this leave you in your search for a good-quality ginger product? I suggest two options:

1. Buy fresh ginger from your local vegetable store or supermarket, or dried ginger in whole hands from an ethnic grocery store. If you buy dried ginger, you can grind it at home in a coffee grinder or with a mortar and pestle.

2. Buy medicinal ginger tablets at your local health food store. If you choose to do this, you should look for a product marketed by a reputable company. A good ginger product may contain ground ginger or ginger extract. Both are effective, although extract is more concentrated. Unquestionably, the best product is standardized—that is, guaranteed by analysis to con-

tain a proper level of active ingredients. Since the main active ingredients in ginger are gingerols, you should look at the package label for a promise that the product contains a given level of gingerols.

There is a third option—purchasing ground ginger from a food store. This is the least advisable option, however, because of the problems with ground spices described above. However, if you have no choice, try at least to purchase the ground ginger from an ethnic grocery store rather than a supermarket, since the ethnic community may be more discriminating than the locals when it comes to the quality of ginger.

DOSAGE

In Oriental medicine, ginger, in its dry form, is given at a dose of 3 grams minimum to 10 grams maximum per day. This is higher than what is recommended for home treatment in the West. Rather, this is what is used by professionals such as herbalists for the treatment of health problems.

Nonprofessionals, and especially the inexperienced, are advised to use dried ginger in doses of 1 gram, or about ⅕ to ¼ teaspoon. This corresponds to a 100-milligram tablet of concentrated ginger extract in pill form. In the case of fresh ginger, the equivalent dose is about 4 grams, or 1 level teaspoon. You can take up to four doses per day as necessary.

For ginger extract, it is difficult to give precise dosage guidelines without having the product in hand because extracts are prepared in a number of different ways. The best advice is to follow the manufacturer's recommendations. The amount you use per dose should be equivalent to 1 gram of dried ginger. The packaging should contain a note describing the equivalent of the recommended dose in terms of ground ginger.

In the *British Pharmacopoeia* of 1973, an alcoholic extract called Strong Ginger Tincture is described. This extract is prepared by steeping 500 grams ground ginger in 1 liter (about 1 quart) of 90-percent alcohol. The dose is given as a half-milliliter (⅒ teaspoon), which is equivalent to only ¼ gram ginger, a very low dose for therapeutic purposes. However, the dose is so low because the tincture was used by pharmacists more for flavoring than as a medicine. In *Martindale's Extra Pharmacopoeia* (London: National Pharmaceutical Union, 1966), the dosage is given as ¼ to 1 gram.

MAKING GINGER MEDICINAL PREPARATIONS

The following recipes are for the more common medicinal preparations featuring ginger. They treat the simple complaints that most people usually do not bring to a doctor anyway.

Ginger Oil

Ginger oil is a very useful remedy for headaches, painful joints, and achy muscles. Make it by mixing 1 part juice of grated ginger with 5 parts sesame oil. To apply, just rub the mixture into the painful area. You can also use ginger oil to treat an earache by putting one or two drops on a cotton ball and placing the cotton ball in the aching ear.

Ginger Compress and Ginger Bath

Put 100 grams (20 teaspoons) finely grated fresh ginger in a piece of cheesecloth. Tie the cheesecloth into a bundle and lower it into a bowl containing 1 quart water that is hot but not boiling. Keep the water at this temperature until it turns yellow, reheating it if necessary.

For a ginger compress, soak a towel in the ginger water and apply the towel repeatedly to the skin. Keep the water and the towel as hot as you can bear. When the liquid cools down, warm it again. The compress has done its job when the skin has turned red, since the redness is a sign that the circulation in the area has been stimulated. A ginger compress is useful for pains, swellings, inflammations, joint problems, and even some internal conditions, especially bronchial problems.

For a ginger bath, add the above ginger water to your bath water. A ginger bath is useful for the same purposes as a ginger compress is, but its effects are much milder, since the ginger water is diluted in the bath water.

Ginger Poultice and Ginger Plaster

Poultices are warm, moist pastes of herbs and other powders that are placed on the skin to relieve inflammations, boils and eruptions, and bites and stings. A poultice of plantain, comfrey, or marshmallow can draw out toxins and heal infections; a poultice of catnip, lobelia, or echinacea can relieve pain and cramps. Ginger can be added to any of these poultices to improve the circulation in the affected area and to help the other herb get inside and do its job.

A ginger plaster, consisting of a paste made of grated ginger mixed with bread or tofu and tied inside a piece of muslin, can be placed on the skin to relieve local inflammations and to draw out fever. A very effective poultice to relieve pain and inflammation and to promote circulation in rheumatic and arthritic conditions was developed by

Michael Tierra, herb expert and author of *Planetary Herbology* (Santa Fe, New Mexico: Lotus Press, 1989). This poultice is made of 2 parts dried ginger root, 1 part cayenne pepper, and ½ part lobelia.

Laxative Mixture

Laxatives such as senna, cascara, and rhubarb root are quite strong. They may cause stomach cramps or pains, or reduce the effective functioning of the digestive system. Therefore, if you take such a laxative, add about 1 part ginger to 2 parts of the laxative to protect the digestion. This is not necessary with bulk-forming laxatives such as flax seed (linseed) or psyllium. Other aromatic carminatives, such as fennel and aniseed, may also be helpful.

Pharmacists' Laxative

Pharmacists use a laxative mixture that contains rhubarb, peppermint, ginger, and gentian. This is a sensible mixture because it combines the laxative element rhubarb with ginger, to improve digestion and remove nausea; peppermint, to prevent cramps and pain; and gentian, to stimulate the appetite and the liver.

The following recipe is from *Martindale's Extra Pharmacopoeia*. It utilizes a strong ginger tincture, made of 50 grams (10 teaspoons) dried ginger steeped in 100 milliliters (3 ½ ounces) alcohol. To make the recipe, combine 3 drops of the ginger tincture with ½ gram sodium bicarbonate, 1 drop peppermint oil, 12 drops concentrated rhubarb infusion, 10 drops concentrated compound gentian infusion, and 3 teaspoons water (chloroform water, according to the printed recipe). This makes one dose.

Chinese Warming Formula

Chinese formulas are individually designed to take into account the specific imbalances that led to the ailment in the particular individual. Therefore, it is hard to give a general formula appropriate for everyone. Instead, you should obtain a prescription from a professional Oriental medical practitioner for a mixture formulated especially for you.

Ginger-Miso Revival Soup

Ginger-Miso Revival Soup aids recuperation from illness and also serves as a nutritious and warming soup during illness. To make it, dissolve 1 level teaspoon miso in 1 cup hot water or, better, vegetable stock. Add a dash of good shoyu sauce, chop in some leeks, and grate in about 2 grams fresh ginger, or a piece about the size of a sugar cube.

Trikatu

Trikatu is the classic Ayurvedic recipe for the digestive system. It is used for nausea, indigestion, poor appetite, colic, gas, candida, coughs and colds, and poor circulation. It is also used to remove toxins. Trikatu is better for Kapha and Vata constitutions and types of problems than for Pitta types (see Chapter 3).

To make Trikatu, combine equal parts ginger, black pepper, and long pepper (*Piper longum*), either as a powder or mixed with honey in the Ayurvedic fashion and formed into pills. The dose is 1 to 3 grams taken two to three times a day. To make this formula gentler, especially for children, replace the long pepper with aniseed. Or, add coriander, nutmeg, or celery seed to enrich the formula and make it milder.

Tea for Cramps and Spasms

Cramp bark is a useful herb for cramps and spasms, just as its name suggests. Michael Tierra has proposed that a tea made of 1 part ginger and 2 parts cramp bark is the optimal mixture. An alternative mixture is equal parts ginger and chamomile. These ginger teas go well with the ginger compress just described.

Ginger Tea for Fevers and Colds

Ginger tea is a classic standby to encourage sweating and to bring out low-grade fevers and colds (see Chapter 4). To make ginger tea, grate a small piece (about 1 gram, or a piece about the size of half a sugar cube) of fresh ginger into an average-size glass or cup. Squeeze in the juice of half a lemon, fill the glass or cup with hot water, and sweeten the tea with a little honey.

Yogi Tea

This recipe is the classic Indian warming tea, nutritive, digestive, calming, and clearing to the mind and body. It is taken by Indian mountain people to warm up and to revive the spirits. To make Yogi Tea, add 2 teaspoons grated fresh ginger, 4 whole cardamoms, 8 whole cloves, and 1 stick cinnamon to 8 cups water. Boil the mixture until it is reduced by half, then add ½ cup milk.

Ayurvedic Tea for Colds

This tea is a classic Indian remedy for colds, catarrh, and congestion, as well as for a beginning flu or other viral illness. It helps the immunity and warms the body.

To make the tea, combine a grated 1-inch piece of ginger, chopped 1-inch piece of licorice, 5 whole peppercorns, and 10 leaves of toolsi, which is Indian holy basil (substitute sweet basil if toolsi is unavailable). Add 2 cups water and boil until the liquid is reduced by half.

HOW SAFE IS GINGER?

We can assume that ginger is very safe indeed. After all, it is a food substance used all over the world in breakfast, lunch, and dinner recipes. It is on the spice shelves of most supermarkets. And it does not carry a health warning on the label. Nevertheless, it is worth checking scientifically.

Research has confirmed ginger's safety. Animals have been given ginger on a daily basis in amounts equivalent to a human's consumption of about 7 ½ pounds without noticeable side effects. When animals are fed pure gingerol or shogaol, they can tolerate amounts equivalent to a human's consumption of about 4 ½ pounds dried ginger.

An extensive survey of the world medical literature has failed to come up with reports of side effects from taking ginger as a food or a medicine and none are given in the pharmacopoeias, the national drug guides, that mention ginger. Indeed, the United States Food and Drug Administration has classified ginger among the safest of herbs, in the Generally Recognized as Safe (GRAS) category. This allows it to be on open and general sale.

Therefore, we know that ginger is completely safe. However, we should also be aware that even the safest food taken in the wrong way can produce adverse effects. Carrots are safe, but too much carrot juice can cause a vitamin A overdose, especially in an individual with a liver problem. In the same vein, ginger should not be taken by a person with a high fever. In addition, if other symptoms of hot conditions are present, ginger is not recommended. Such symptoms include dryness with a rapid pulse, red skin, a bright red tongue, dehydration, and blood in the stool. These conditions do not turn ginger into a raging poison, but ginger could accentuate the symptoms of over-heating.

CHAPTER 9

Ginger Up
Your Cooking

Ginger is a symbol of the merging of the kitchen cupboard with the medicine cabinet. In a holistic sense, the entire field of medicine needs to be brought back into the mainstream of life. By that I mean that it needs to be rejoined with our world as a normal, natural influence, with no essential difference seen between a pitcher of clean water that satisfies thirst and a mug of herbal tea that treats a potential health problem.

From that perspective, there is nothing wrong with cooking with our medicines and nothing incorrect about including recipes for lunch in a book on herbal remedies. This chapter will therefore look at some of the ways in which ginger can be included in our normal diet. Of course, this is not a cookbook, so the recipes will be samples rather than full menus.

As I mentioned in Chapter 1, the amounts of ginger and other spices included in recipes for food dishes are not sufficient to cure ailments. But these spices do have a range of gentle and long-term health benefits such as

warming the body, clearing out toxins, promoting digestion and elimination, improving absorption of nutrients,
preventing food poisoning and rancidity, and helping prevent atherosclerosis. In other words, cooking with medicinal foods like ginger, garlic, aniseed, linseed, fenugreek,
mustard, cinnamon, caraway, thyme, and mint will generally have a preventive rather than curative health role.

MAIN DISHES

Ginger is a classic addition to meat and poultry dishes
throughout Asia, particularly because it helps to predigest
and absorb meat. It should be even more important these
days because the health status of factory-farmed, pesti-
cide-loaded meat and poultry seems dire. I, myself, have
been a vegetarian for many years, so I cannot claim famili-
arity with cooking these items. However, I am so familiar
with the use of spices, especially after two years in India,
that I feel safe in recommending one or two ideas.

All steaks will benefit from being rubbed all over with
fresh ginger before and during braising or grilling. So will
chicken. For example, before roasting a chicken, rub it all
over with a paste made of a 2-inch piece of fresh ginger,
crushed; 2 garlic cloves, crushed; and salt.

Ginger is also one of the secrets of Oriental fish dishes.
It gives a delicate and aromatic flavor to fish and makes
the dish light and easy to digest. You must take care not to
overcook the ginger or the fish, however.

The following recipes will show you how to make dishes
that are both delicious and nutritious. These dishes reflect
a wide range of international cuisines that incorporate the
distinct taste of ginger. They have all been thoroughly
kitchen-tested. Whether you are a beginning cook or an
experienced chef, you will find these recipes complete and
easy to follow.

Chicken Chow Mein

This is a classic Chinese dish that needs its ginger.

Yield: 3 servings

7 ounces chicken pieces
1 cup chicken stock
7 ounces uncooked egg noodles
½ cup vegetable oil
½ medium head of cabbage, cored and shredded
2 ounces mushrooms, sliced
2 leeks, sliced
1-inch piece fresh ginger, chopped
2 garlic cloves, crushed
2 teaspoons vinegar
2 teaspoons shoyu sauce
2 teaspoons tomato sauce
1 teaspoon chili sauce
Margarine
2 eggs, beaten

1. In a medium-size skillet, simmer the chicken in the chicken stock for about 15 minutes. Remove the chicken from the stock and set the stock aside. When the chicken has cooled enough to be comfortably handled, shred it and set it aside.

2. In a medium-size saucepan, cook the noodles according to the package directions. Drain, rinse, and return to the pot.

3. In a large heavy-bottom pot or a wok, heat the vegetable oil over medium heat. Add the cabbage, mushrooms, leeks, ginger, garlic, and shredded chicken; sauté for 3 to 4 minutes, stirring constantly. Add the cooked noodles and stir-fry for an additional minute. Add the reserved chicken stock, vinegar, shoyu sauce, tomato sauce, and chili sauce; stir. Transfer to a serving platter and keep warm.

4. In a small skillet, melt some margarine over low heat. Add half of the beaten egg and cook into a small, flat

omelette. Remove from the skillet, roll up, slice, and add to the chicken-vegetable mixture as a garnish. Repeat with the remaining beaten egg. Serve immediately.

Chinese Ginger Fish

This is a simple recipe for a Chinese-style fish dish.

Yield: 3–4 servings

1 pound white fish fillets
¼ cup sherry
4 leeks, sliced
½ teaspoon ground ginger
¼–½ teaspoon salt
3 tablespoons sesame oil
¼ teaspoon coarsely ground black pepper
½ lemon, sliced, as garnish

1. In a small baking dish, arrange the fish fillets in a single layer. In a small bowl, combine the sherry, leeks, ground ginger, and salt; drizzle over the fish. Let the fish marinate for 1 hour, then remove from the dish, reserving the marinade.

2. In a medium-size heavy-bottom skillet, heat the sesame oil over medium heat. Add the marinated fish and fry until browned on both sides, about 5 minutes. Add the reserved marinade and continue cooking briefly, for less than 1 minute.

3. To serve, sprinkle the fish with the black pepper and garnish with the lemon slices.

Chinese Ginger Steak

This recipe is for a typical Chinese ginger steak.

Yield: 5–6 servings

2 tablespoons sesame oil
2 onions, sliced, with slices halved
2 garlic cloves, crushed
2-inch piece fresh ginger, finely chopped
2 pounds rump roast or sirloin steak, cut into slivers
2 tablespoons shoyu sauce
¼ teaspoon salt
¼ teaspoon coarsely ground black pepper
2 cups water

1. In a medium-size saucepan, heat the sesame oil over medium heat. Add the onions and garlic, and sauté until golden brown, about 3 minutes.

2. Add the ginger and cook for an additional 1 to 2 minutes.

3. Stir in the meat, shoyu sauce, salt, black pepper, and water. Raise the heat to high and bring the mixture to a boil, then cover, reduce the heat, and simmer until the meat is tender, about 20 minutes. Serve immediately.

VEGETABLE DISHES

Indian dishes often contain ginger in the *masala*, which is a mixture of spices used for cooking. In some regions, particularly in colder areas, ginger is the dominant note. Very often, meat and vegetables are transposable in Indian cooking, with the same basic procedure used for each.

Try adding ground ginger to rice that has just finished cooking. Both cinnamon and ginger add an aromatic zest to plain rice. Rice can also be enriched by being cooked with cinnamon sticks, nuts, raisins, and a bay leaf or two,

which you can add with the cold water at the beginning.
Sprinkle the cooked rice with ginger before serving.

Channa Masala (Spiced Chickpeas)

This is one of my favorite dishes.

Yield: 4–5 servings

9 ounces dried chickpeas
1 tablespoon mango powder
1 teaspoon ground cumin
1 teaspoon ground coriander
½ teaspoon chili powder
½ teaspoon salt
2 teaspoons garam masala
1 red or green sweet pepper, chopped
2-inch piece fresh ginger, grated
¼ cup vegetable oil
or ghee (Indian-style clarified butter)

1. The night before, place the chickpeas in a large bowl. Add water to cover and let soak overnight.

2. The next day, transfer the chickpeas and water to a large saucepan. Bring to a boil over high heat, then reduce the heat and simmer until the chickpeas are soft, about 1 hour. Strain the chickpeas and reserve the liquid.

3. In a clean large bowl, combine the drained chickpeas with the mango powder, cumin, coriander, red chili powder, and salt; toss. Sprinkle with the garam masala and add the sweet peppers and ginger; toss again.

4. In a medium-size saucepan, heat the vegetable oil or ghee over medium heat. Add the chickpea mixture and sauté for 5 minutes, adding the reserved chickpea liquid a few teaspoonfuls at a time and stirring constantly. Serve immediately.

Ginger Vegetable

Ginger goes very well with a single vegetable cooked in butter or ghee. The following recipe is an example.

Yield: 3–4 servings

¼ cup butter or ghee
1 medium head cauliflower (about 2 pounds), broken
into small florets
2-inch piece fresh ginger, thinly sliced
¼ teaspoon salt
¼ teaspoon coarsely ground black pepper

1. In a medium-size saucepan, melt the butter or ghee over low heat. Add the cauliflower, ginger, and salt. Cover and cook until the cauliflower is tender, about 10 minutes.

2. To serve, sprinkle with the black pepper.

Matar Aloo

This is a simple classic household curry of northern India.

Yield: 4 servings

1/4 cup vegetable oil or ghee
1 medium onion, sliced
2-inch piece fresh ginger, sliced
1 cup yogurt or puréed tomatoes
1 pound potatoes, cut into 1/2-inch cubes
7 ounces fresh or frozen peas
1/2 teaspoon ground cumin
1/2 teaspoon ground coriander
1/4–1/2 teaspoon chili powder
1/2 teaspoon salt
1/3 teaspoon turmeric powder
Coriander leaves, as garnish

1. In a large saucepan, heat the vegetable oil or ghee over medium heat. Add the onions and ginger, and sauté until the onions have softened and are beginning to brown, about 5 to 7 minutes.

2. Add the yogurt or tomatoes, and sauté for an additional 3 to 4 minutes.

3. Add the potatoes, peas, cumin, coriander, chili powder, salt, and turmeric powder. Cook gently, stirring constantly, for 2 minutes more.

4. Add water to cover and raise the heat to high. Bring to a boil, then cover, reduce the heat, and simmer until the potatoes are tender, about 10 minutes.

5. To serve, garnish with the coriander leaves.

Ginger Sweet Potatoes

Some vegetables can be cooked, sweetened, or glazed with ginger. Sweet potatoes are just one example.

Yield: 3–4 servings

4 medium sweet potatoes, sliced
¼ teaspoon salt
¼ teaspoon freshly ground black pepper
2 tablespoons butter
½ cup orange juice
2 tablespoons honey
¾ teaspoon ground ginger

1. Preheat the oven to 375°F.

2. In a medium-size saucepan, place the sweet potato slices in water to cover. Bring to a boil over high heat, then reduce the heat and simmer until the sweet potatoes are soft, about 15 to 20 minutes.

3. Lightly grease a medium-size casserole dish. Line the bottom of the dish with one layer of sweet potato slices, then sprinkle the sweet potatoes with some of the salt and black pepper. Dot with some of the butter. Repeat layering until all the sweet potato slices are used.

4. In a small bowl, mix the orange juice, honey, and ground ginger. Pour over the sweet potatoes. Place the casserole dish in the oven and bake for about 20 to 30 minutes. Serve hot.

Variation

For a less-sweet glaze, omit the honey and substitute the juice of 1 lemon for the orange juice.

CHUTNEYS AND PICKLES

Chutneys and pickles are favorite items in India. The following recipes should make them popular in your house, too.

Carrot Pickles

*A carrot pickle is cheap and easy to make
and also needs its ginger.*

Yield: About 7 cups

2 pounds carrots, trimmed and peeled
1 teaspoon salt
1 cup chopped green or red sweet pepper
6 garlic cloves, minced
2 tablespoons ground mustard seed
1 tablespoon coarsely ground pepper
2 teaspoons cumin seeds
2 teaspoons ground ginger
Cider vinegar

1. If the carrots are large, slice them or cut them into chunks. If the carrots are small, leave them whole. Place the carrots in a large saucepan containing about 2 inches of water and bring them to a boil over high heat. Then cover the saucepan, reduce the heat, and simmer until the carrots are partially cooked, about 5 minutes. Drain the carrots, sprinkle them with the salt, and let them sit, covered, for 24 hours.

2. The next day, add the sweet peppers, garlic, ground mustard seed, ground peppercorns, cumin seed, and ground ginger. Add just enough cider vinegar to cover everything. Let sit for about 3 days.

3. After 3 days, check the carrots. They are done if they have softened and become spicy in taste. Transfer them to airtight jars.

Ginger Pickles

*This is one of the best ginger pickles I have ever tasted
and is also the simplest to make.
A few slices will add fireworks to any meal.*

**Fresh ginger, thinly sliced
Cider vinegar**

1. In a glass jar, combine the ginger slices with just enough cider vinegar to cover.

2. Place the jar in the sun and let stand for 10 days.

Ginger Chutney

This is a traditional Indian ginger chutney.

Yield: 3 cups

1–2 tablespoons mustard oil or sesame oil
2 tablespoons mustard seeds
14-ounce piece fresh ginger, crushed
10 ounces garlic cloves, crushed
1 ⅛ cups vinegar
1 cup brown sugar
2 teaspoons chili powder
2 teaspoons salt
1 teaspoon cumin seeds

1. In a large saucepan, heat the mustard oil or sesame oil over medium heat. Add the mustard seeds and cook until the seeds begin to pop.

2. Add the ginger, garlic, vinegar, brown sugar, chili powder, salt, and cumin seeds. Stir, reduce the heat, and cook gently until the ginger and garlic are soft. Remove from the heat and let cool.

3. When the chutney has cooled, pour it into jars.

Coconut Chutney

*Everyone who visits southern India falls in love with the
fresh coconut chutneys. The following is a simple recipe.*

Yield: 2 cups

1 cup grated fresh coconut
1-inch piece fresh ginger, chopped
1 heaping tablespoon chopped coriander leaves
1 small green chili, trimmed, seeded, and chopped
½ teaspoon salt
Juice of 1 lemon or lime, or ½ cup yogurt

1. In a large bowl, combine the coconut and ginger. Stir
in the coriander, chili, and salt. Add the lemon or lime
juice or the yogurt, and mix into a paste. Place in the
refrigerator for at least 2 hours.
2. Serve chilled.

Tomato Chutney

*Tomatoes prepared this way will add drama to any dish.
It is what ketchup aspires to but never can reach!*

Yield: 3 cups

6 medium tomatoes
Rind of 1 large lemon or lime, grated
2-inch piece fresh ginger, grated
1 teaspoon coarsely ground black pepper
¼ teaspoon chopped basil leaves
¼ teaspoon paprika
¼ teaspoon turmeric

1. In a large saucepan, boil the tomatoes in water to
cover until soft, about 15 minutes.
2. Drain the tomatoes and pound gently into pulp. Place
the pulp in a large bowl and add the lemon or lime
rind, ginger, black pepper, basil, paprika, and tur-

meric; mix well. Place in the refrigerator for at least 2 hours.

3. Serve chilled.

DESSERTS AND SNACKS

Ginger, like cinnamon, goes well with baked fruit and all kinds of desserts. It adds both aroma and a little extra pungency. Stem ginger—that is, sweet preserved ginger (see page 64)—has always been used in desserts. However, it has little of its original pungent and aromatic constituents left.

Grapefruit tastes sublime when sprinkled with a mixture of brown sugar or honey and ginger. The same goes for melon, which also requires some lemon juice for tartness. There are many popular desserts, snacks, and other sweet items featuring ginger. The following recipes are just a sampling.

Ginger Ice Cream

This is one of the fringe flavors of ice cream
that has its devoted followers.

Yield: 3–4 servings

5 ounces ginger syrup
2–3 ounces preserved ginger, chopped
1 teaspoon ground ginger
1 ¼ cups cream, partially whipped
¾ cup prepared custard, any flavor
¼ cup superfine sugar

1. In a large bowl, mix together the ginger syrup, preserved ginger, and ground ginger. Fold in the cream,
   custard, and sugar. Pour into a plastic container and
   place in the refrigerator until chilled. When chilled,
   transfer to the freezer for about 2 hours.

2. Remove the frozen mixture from the freezer and beat
   by hand or with an electric mixer to break up the ice
   crystals. Return to the freezer until frozen again,
   about 2 hours more.

Variation

For a lighter ice cream, substitute 2 beaten egg whites for
the custard.

Ginger Pumpkin Pie

While backpacking through Nepal in 1975, I enjoyed
"the best pumpkin pie this side of the Atlantic Ocean"
in a teahouse at a crossroads near the little town of
Dhulikel, which sits along the Chinese border.
I am convinced that fresh green mountain ginger
contributed to the pie's magnificence. While I never got the
exact recipe, I have approximated it as follows.

Yield: 16 servings

2 ½ cups all-purpose flour
1 cup sugar
1 ¾-ounce piece fresh ginger, grated
1 teaspoon baking powder
1 teaspoon baking soda
1 teaspoon salt
¾ teaspoon cinnamon
¼ teaspoon ground cloves
1 ½ cups puréed boiled pumpkin
1 cup brown sugar
½ cup buttermilk
7 tablespoons butter or vegetable shortening
3 eggs, beaten

1. Preheat the oven to 350°F. Grease and flour two 9-inch-diameter flan tins.

2. In a large bowl, sift together the flour, sugar, ginger, baking powder, baking soda, salt, cinnamon, and cloves. Add the pumpkin, brown sugar, buttermilk, and butter or shortening; beat briefly. Add the eggs and beat again.

3. Pour the batter into the flan tins and place the tins in the oven. Bake until the pies are firm, about 45 minutes. Let cool before serving.

Light Ginger Pumpkin Pie

This is the recipe I now use to make pumpkin pie.
It is a light version of that wonderful pie
I savored in Nepal.

Yield: 8 servings

2 cups puréed boiled pumpkin
2 tablespoons tahini (sesame paste)
½ teaspoon cinnamon
½ teaspoon ground ginger or
1-inch piece fresh ginger, grated
¼ teaspoon ground cloves
Honey to taste
1 prepared 9-inch pie crust
Nuts and raisins, as garnish

1. Preheat the oven to 350°F.
2. In a large bowl, combine the pumpkin, tahini, cinnamon, ginger, cloves, and honey; mix well. Pour into the pie crust.
3. Decorate the pie with the nuts and raisins, if desired.
4. Place the pie in the oven and bake until the filling is firm, about 30 minutes. Let cool before serving.

Variation

Use a pie shell with nuts and raisins baked in.

Pumpkin Bread

*This recipe is not only a favorite of mine
but is also popular with my family and friends.*

Yield: 24 servings

3 cups whole-wheat flour
1 teaspoon baking soda
½ teaspoon salt
2 cups water
1 ½ cups puréed boiled pumpkin
1 egg, beaten
1-inch piece of fresh ginger, grated
½ teaspoon cinnamon
¼ teaspoon nutmeg
¼ teaspoon ground cloves
⅓ cup raisins
⅓ cup chopped walnuts and/or cashew nuts

1. Preheat the oven to 400°F. Oil a 13-x-9-inch cake pan.

2. In a large bowl, combine the flour, baking soda, salt, and water. Add the pumpkin and egg, and stir. Add the ginger, cinnamon, nutmeg, and cloves; stir again. Fold in the raisins and nuts. If necessary, add more flour or water to correct the consistency of the batter. Pour into the cake pan.

3. Place the cake in the oven and bake until a toothpick inserted in the center comes out clean, about 45 minutes.

Gingerbread Men

*This is my personal recipe for healthy,
holistic gingerbread men.*

Yield: About 8 large men or 24 small men

½ cup vegetable oil or melted butter
½ cup honey
½ cup water
2 cups whole-wheat flour
2 teaspoons ground ginger
1 teaspoon salt
½ teaspoon ground cloves
½ teaspoon cinnamon
½ teaspoon allspice
Decorations such as currants, raisins, and nuts

1. Preheat the oven to 350°F.

2. In a large bowl, mix together the vegetable oil or melted butter, the honey, and the water. Stir in just enough flour to make a thick batter. Add the ginger, salt, cloves, cinnamon, and allspice; mix well. Add additional flour if necessary to make a stiff dough. Cover the bowl and place in the refrigerator for about 30 minutes.

3. When the dough is chilled, remove it from the refrigerator and turn it out onto a floured surface. Roll it out to ¼-inch thick. Using a cardboard stencil or cookie cutter if necessary, cut out little man shapes. Decorate using the currants, raisins, and nuts for the eyes, noses, buttons, and so on. Place the cookies on a cookie sheet.

4. Place the cookies in the oven and bake until firm, about 15 minutes. Let cool on cookie sheet before serving.

BEVERAGES

The wise host always has homemade ginger beverages on hand. Ginger wine and ginger punch are traditional drinks for loosening up yourself and your guests on chilly evenings, while ginger ale is wonderful alone or as a mixer.

Ginger Ale

Ginger ale is available in bottles and cans as a debilitated, saccharined soft drink. If you want to taste the real thing, with the real taste of ginger, try this recipe.

Yield: 5 quarts

2 ½ cups sugar
1-ounce piece fresh ginger, well crushed
1 heaping teaspoon cream of tartar
1 gallon boiling water
Juice and rinds of 2 large lemons
1 teaspoon dry beer yeast

1. In a large bowl, combine the sugar, ginger, and cream of tartar. Pour in the boiling water and stir. Let cool.

2. When the mixture has cooled, add the lemon juice, lemon rinds, and yeast. Cover the bowl, set it in a warm place, and let the mixture ferment for 3 days. Check the mixture periodically and skim off any yeast that rises to the surface.

3. When the mixture has fermented, strain or siphon it into bottles. Do not cap the bottles too tightly. Let the mixture stand another week at room temperature before serving.

Ginger Wine

Ginger wine is wonderful on a cold night.
It is a great digestive aid as well.

Yield: 3 ½ quarts

> 1 packet dry yeast or dry wine yeast
> 1 gallon warm water
> 7 ½ cups sugar
> Juice and rinds of 2 large lemons
> Juice and rinds of 2 large oranges
> 2-ounce piece fresh ginger, grated
> ¼ teaspoon cayenne pepper
> 3 cups raisins, chopped
> 1 packet yeast nutrient
> (available in wine making stores)

1. In a small jar, proof the dry yeast or dry wine yeast by combining it with ½ cup of the warm water and 2 teaspoons of the sugar. Let it stand for 1 to 2 hours.

2. In a large saucepan, combine the lemon rinds, orange rinds, ginger, cayenne pepper, and remaining water. Bring to a boil over high heat. Remove from the heat and add the remaining sugar, stirring until dissolved. Add the raisins and let the mixture cool.

3. When the mixture has cooled, add the lemon juice, orange juice, proofed yeast, and yeast nutrient. Set the bowl in a warm place and let the mixture ferment for 1 week.

4. After 1 week, strain the liquid and press the raisins. Put the liquid in a bottle with an airlock to let out the gases and to continue to ferment for another 2 weeks.

5. After 2 weeks, check the wine. It should be still and not exhibit any gassing. Allow it to stand until clear, about 2 weeks more.

6. Siphon the wine into bottles and serve.

Ginger Punch

*This is a spiced alcoholic, or partially alcoholic, drink
that absolutely requires ginger along with the clear,
astringent aroma of cloves.*

Yield: 2 ½ quarts

2 bottles red wine
½ cup brown sugar
1 pint rum
1 pint orange juice
1 pint apple juice
2-inch piece fresh ginger, crushed
1 teaspoon crumbled cinnamon stick
6 whole cloves
Juice and rinds of 1–2 lemons

1. In a large saucepan, combine the wine, brown sugar, rum, orange juice, apple juice, ginger, cinnamon, and cloves. Add the lemon rinds and warm gently over low heat; do not boil.

2. When ready to serve, stir in the lemon juice.

Hopefully, from the representative recipes in this chapter, you have had your appetite whetted enough so that you will be on the lookout for additional recipes containing ginger. The process of cooking is an alchemy, as is the preparation of medicines. It blends qualities and elements from nature to achieve a satisfying effect on us. One way or another, it is ginger's natural destination.

CHAPTER 10

Conclusion

Despite the previous chapter's devotion to desserts and drinks, the main purpose of this book is to teach the reader to take ginger more seriously. During the twentieth century, ginger has been in a pickle in more ways than one. Relegating ginger to the back of the spice shelf, letting it get old and dried, and ignoring it in family health care, we have all but lost the knowledge of how to employ it. Ginger has become something used in ginger ale and ginger steak, and it seems incredible to us that lengthy and sophisticated treatises are written in Oriental medicine and Indian traditional medicine about how best to use ginger to heal all kinds of conditions, some of them serious.

But we can now begin to see that we have been ignorant. A seemingly endless knowledge exists of how to use ginger in health care and for the prevention and treatment of a wide variety of ailments. This knowledge starts with straightforward information on the properties of the plant and its uses in treating specific health problems, and moves on to a study of its constituents. It then goes on to a look at what other remedies ginger is classified with based on its therapeutic uses and chemical constituents, and to the connections between ginger and these remedies. It continues with the more subtle art of knowing how best to use the plant for its energetic qualities—that is, for its healing, cooling, energizing, moving, stimulating, and other effects—and how these qualities work in the different organ systems of the body. There is also the deep knowledge of how different kinds of people, manifesting health problems in different ways, should use ginger. Finally, there is the ancient knowledge of how the herb combines in mixtures with other herbs, so that each herb complements the others, in special combinations designed for individual health situations.

All this just about ginger. And consider that there are several thousand other herbal and mineral remedies to learn about. Readers of this book will no longer, I hope, take the attitude that ginger and other spices are irrelevant and uninteresting, fit only for perking up the occasional curry.

So, the potential knowledge is immense. No wonder an Oriental herbalist has to study for fifty years before he is recognized as a true master of his trade. This may sound rather daunting or discouraging. Who can grasp all this information? Does everyone have to study for fifty years before being considered capable of treating a cold?

Today, few people indeed are alive who are true masters in that sense. Instead, aspects of herbal information are being avidly collected by more modern-minded herbalists and researchers. In addition, a groundswell of interest is building among the general population, with more people every day wanting to learn simple, useful measures that will enable them to have and use a well-stocked herbal first-aid kit. In other words, all of us are somewhat in between the master herbalist and the innocent questioner who is amazed that one can write, or even read, a whole book on ginger. Having a good store of information on ginger, perhaps more than one person can ever use, increases the general network of herbal lore within our culture, creating a kind of invisible archive of health-care practices that can be drawn on more and more.

TAKING IT HOME

Now that you have read this whole book on ginger, you can choose to ignore ginger as another faddish health-care curiosity. Or, you can choose to see ginger as useful only to those strange folk who have the time to mess around with things like ginger compresses. Or, you can decide to take ginger now and then for an occasional stomachache or winter chill. Or, you can go whole hog and treat ginger as a new discovery that opens up other dimensions of self-care and holistic living.

If this last possibility seems a bit far-fetched, then let us look again at the main uses for ginger that we have discussed. Ginger is the best-known remedy for nausea, vomiting, and stomach upsets, ills that we all experience at times. It has an important use for a variety of other digestive disturbances, from indigestion to constipation. It stimulates the circulation, bringing warmth and life back into cold and congested body systems. It stimulates the heart and thins the blood. It helps to treat chronic low-grade infections and fevers. It helps to warm the lungs and chest and to get rid of colds, catarrh, and bronchial problems. It reduces toxicity, burns up poisons in the body, and aids rheumatic and menstrual disturbances. In addition, it helps with the absorption of foods and other medicines.

The power of ginger continues with its culinary uses.

Besides bringing an aromatic vitality to a multitude of foods and drinks, it helps the digestion and absorption of the foods it accompanies, acts as an antioxidant, purifies the body of any toxins that might have crept in with food, reduces the amount of cholesterol being absorbed by the body, and protects the stomach.

All this is quite remarkable from a single medicinal food. And consider that ginger is only one of a number of medicinal foods that you can find in the average kitchen, each of which may have a similar range of potential uses. Garlic, onion, turmeric, cayenne pepper, mint, and fenugreek are all examples. All these foods offer a window—a kitchen window—of opportunity into a whole world of considerable interest and vitality.

The more we use herbs and spices, and the more we know about them, the farther we go into a fascinating world where we relate much more fully to the things we consume. We learn how to gain better health and well-being. We become busy in all kinds of internal experiments, much like the ancient alchemists, trying out exactly when and how different herbs and medicinal foods help us. We experience a kaleidoscope of tastes and aromas in our cooking and handling of foods. Above all, we gain extra control over our lives; we can design and use our own flavors and medicines, which can be a source of great joy and security.

This last statement needs some explanation. When you go to the doctor—say with chronic bronchitis or angina pectoris or high blood pressure—you put yourself in the hands of a professional. He uses a language and techniques that you know nothing about, prescribes medications whose names you possibly cannot pronounce. You become a patient, and you begin to feel like one. In a subtle way, you lose control over the most important thing in your life, namely your health and feeling of well-being. On the other hand, if you get busy working on yourself, using some of the natural aids that are all around, you stay out of that dependent category. The same goes for cooking. What you consume has powerful, long-term effects on your health. But most people resign this control to food manufacturers and food processors who cannot be said to have your personal well-being at the forefront of their minds. The result is not only dead and artificial foods that create a vast amount of disease, from allergies to cancer. More than that, a whole vital area of activity is lost from your control, and your life thereby becomes poorer. The few extra minutes it takes to grate ginger and cook real, wholesome foods will return you to yourself and help you to become richly rewarded.

So, get busy with ginger. Add some fresh ginger to your vegetable rack. Put some in your medicine cabinet. Explore some of its uses. Enjoy its possibilities. Then move on to the next herb, and the next spice, and the next.

Further Reading

HERBAL GUIDES

Bensky, D. *Chinese Herbal Medicine: Formulas and Strategies.* Seattle: Eastland Press, 1993.

Fawley, D. *Ayurvedic Healing.* Santa Fe, New Mexico: Morson Press, 1989.

Grieve, M. *A Modern Herbal.* London: Penguin Books, 1976.

Griggs, B. *Green Pharmacy: A History of Herbal Medicine.* Rochester, Vermont: Healing Arts Press, 1990.

Hallowell, Michael. *Herbal Healing.* Garden City Park, New York: Avery Publishing Group, 1994.

Holmes, P. *The Energetics of Western Herbs.* Boulder, Colorado: Artemis Press, POB 1824, 1993.

Mills, S. *Out of the Earth: The Essential Book of Herbal Medicine.* London and New York: Viking, 1992.

Ody, P. *The Herb Society's Complete Medicinal Herbal.* London and New York: Dorling Kindersley, 1993.

Svoboda, R. E. *Ayurveda: Life, Health and Longevity.* London and New York: Viking Penguin, 1992.

Tierra, M. *Planetary Herbology*. Santa Fe, New Mexico: Lotus Press, 1989.

Weiss, R. F. *Herbal Medicine*. Beaconsfield, Buckinghamshire, England: Beaconsfield Publishers, 1988.

GINGER—COOKING

Santa Maria, J. *Indian Vegetarian Cookery*. London: Rider, 1977.

Seely, C. *Ginger Up Your Cookery*. London: Hutchinson Benham, 1982.

GINGER—GENERAL, AGRICULTURE, HISTORY, AND CHEMISTRY

Connell, D. W. "The Chemistry of the Essential Oil and Oleoresin of Ginger (*Zingiber officinale Roscoe*)." *Flavor Industry* 1:677–693 (1970).

Duke, J. "The Joy of Ginger." *American Health*, May 1988.

Govindarajan, V. S. "Ginger—Chemistry, Technology and Quality Evaluation." *CRC Critical Reviews of Food Sciences and Nutrition* 17:1–258 (1982).

Ilyas, M. "The Spices of India." *Economic Botany* 32:238–263 (1978).

Sakamura, F. "Changes in Volatile Constituents of *Zingiber officinale* During Storage." *Phytochemistry* 26:2207–2212 (1987).

GINGER—PHARMACOLOGY AND CLINICAL STUDIES

Al-Yahya, M. A., et al. "Gastroprotective Activity of ginger

Zingiber officinale Rosc., in Rats." *American Journal of Chinese Medicine* 17:51–56 (1989).

Atal, C. K., et al. "Scientific Evidence on the Role of Ayurvedic Herbals on the Bioavailability of Drugs." *Journal of Ethnopharmacology* 4:229–232 (1981).

Bone, M. E., et al. "Ginger in Postoperative Nausea and Vomiting." *Anaesthesia* 45:669–671 (1990).

Fischer-Rasmussen, W., et al. "Ginger Treatment of Hyperemesis Gravidarum." *European Journal of Obstetrics, Gynecology and Reproductive Biology* 38:19–24 (1991).

Grontved, A., and E. Hentzer. "Vertigo-Reducing Effects of Ginger Root." *Journal of Oto-Rhino-Laryngology* 48:282–286 (1986).

Gujral, S., et al. "Effect of Ginger (*Zingiber officinale Roscoe*) Oleoresin on Serum Cholesterol Levels in Cholesterol Fed Rats." *Nutrition Reports International* 17:183–189 (1978).

Mascob, N., et al. "Ethnopharmacological Investigations on Ginger (*Zingiber officinale*)." *Journal of Ethnopharmacology* 27:129–140 (1989).

Mowrey, D. B., and D. E. Claysion. "Motion Sickness, Ginger and Psychophysics." *Lancet* 1:655–657 (1982).

Mustafa, T., and K. C. Srivastava. "Ginger (*Zingiber officinale*) in Migraine Headache." *Journal of Ethnopharmacology* 29:267–273 (1990).

Phillips, S., et al. "*Zingiber officinale* (Ginger): An Antiemetic for Day Case Surgery." *Anaesthesia* 48:715–717 (1993).

Rattan, S. I. "Science Behind the Spices: Inhibition of Platelet Aggregation and Prostaglandin Synthesis." *Bioessays* 8:161–162 (1988).

Shoji, N., et al. "Cardiotonic Principles of Ginger (*Zingiber officinale Roscoe*)." *Journal of Pharmaceutical Sciences* 71:1174–1175 (1982).

Srivastava, K., et al. "Ginger and Rheumatic Disorders." *Medical Hypothesis* 29:25–28 (1989).

GENERAL SELF-CARE

Aihara, Cornellia, and Herman Aihara. *Natural Healing From Head to Toe*. Garden City Park, New York: Avery Publishing Group, 1994.

Balch, James F., and Phyllis A. Balch. *Prescription for Nutritional Healing*. Garden City Park, New York: Avery Publishing Group, 1996.

Bricklin, M. *The Practical Encyclopedia of Natural Healing*. Emmaus, Pennsylvania: Rodale Press, 1993.

Christie, J. *Food for Vitality*. New York: Bantam, 1992.

Collins, J. *Life Forces*. London: New English Library, 1992.

Fulder, S. *How to Survive Medical Treatment*. Saffron Walden, England: C.W. Daniel, 1994.

Northrup, C. *Women's Bodies, Women's Wisdom*. New York: Bantam, 1995.

Pitchford, P. *Healing With Whole Foods*. Berkeley, California: North Atlantic Books, 1993.

Vogel, H.C.A. *The Nature Doctor*. Edinburgh, Scotland: Mainstream, 1994.

Werbach, M. R. *Nutritional Influences on Illness*. Tarzana, California: Third Line Press, 1993.

Index

North America
  ginger consumption in
    modern, 61
  introduction of ginger
    into, 91–92
Nutmeg, 7

Oats, 37
Obesity, ginger's effect on,
    8, 29
Oil of ginger, 69–72, 75,
    99
Oleoresin, 71–72
Onion, 6, 8, 132
Oriental medicine, use of
    ginger in, 11, 17–19, 27,
    33, 34, 38, 42, 46, 49, 51,
    98, 102, 130

Pace, Dr. J.C., 38
Papua New Guinea,
    ginger in, 81
Parsley seed, 50
Pennyroyal, 51
Pepper, 30, 41, 82, 87
  black, 7
  cayenne, 8, 16, 20, 30, 50,
    132
Peppermint, 101
Pharmacopoeias, 9. *See also*
    British Pharmacopoeia;
    Martindale's Extra
    Pharmacopoeia.
Phlai. *See Zingiber cassumu-*
    nar.

Planetary Herbology
    (Tierra), 101
Plantain, 31, 100
Pliny, Gaius, 84–85
Poisons. *See* Toxins.
Pollen, 37
Polo, Marco, 83
Poria, 19
Premenstrual syndrome
    (PMS). *See* Menstrual
    problems.
Preservatives, spices as, 7
Prince of Tai, 82
Prostaglandins, 22, 48,
    75
Protease, 73
Protein, in ginger, 68
Psyllium, 40, 101
Ptolemy, 85
Pumpkin Bread, 123
Pythagoras, 28, 89

Qi, 27

Raspberry leaf, 31
Rheumatic conditions. *See*
    Arthritis.
Rhubarb, 40
Rhubarb root, 101
Romance of the Rose
    (Chaucer), 88
Rome, ancient, spices and,
    84, 90
Rosemary, 6, 7
Rue, 51